ABC of Asthma, Allergies and Lupus

Eradicate Asthma - Now!

A Self-Education Manual for Those Who Prefer
to Adhere to the Logic of the Natural and
the Simple in Preventive Medicine

F. Batmanghelidj, M.D.©
Author of *Your Body's Many Cries for Water*

Global Health Solutions, Inc.
P.O. Box 3189, Falls Church, VA 22043 U.S.A.
Telephone: 703-848-2333 — Fax: 703-848-0028

Website: www.watercure.com

ABC of Asthma, Allergies and Lupus

Copyright © 2000 by F. Batmanghelidj, M.D.
ISBN 0-9629942-6-X

First Edition: August 2000

Global Health Solutions, Inc.
2146 Kings Garden Way
Falls Church, VA 22043
Telephone: 703-848-2333 — Fax: 703-848-0028
Website: *www.watercure.com*

To our **CREATOR**, with awe, humility, dedication and love.

"To tell the truth is not only a responsibility to yourself and others. It is an honor, a duty and your legacy to generations to come. It is a part of their rightful inheritance."

unknown

I thank Caroline Braun for her masterful editorial assistance.

Contents

Disclaimer

The information and recommendations on water intake presented in this book are based on training, personal experience, very extensive research, and other publications of the author on the topic of water metabolism of the body.

The author and producer of this book does not dispense medical advice or prescribe the use or the discontinuance of any medication as a form of treatment without the advice of an attending physician, either directly or indirectly.

The intent of the author, based on the most recent knowledge of micro-anatomy and molecular physiology, is to offer information on the importance of water to well-being, and to help inform the public and medical professionals of the damaging effects of chronic unintentional dehydration to the body, from childhood to old age.

This book is not intended as a replacement for sound medical advice from a physician. On the contrary, sharing of the information contained in this book with the attending physician is highly desirable. Application of the information and recommendations described herein are undertaken at the individual's own risk. The adoption of the information should be in strict compliance with the instructions given herein.

Very sick persons with a past history of major diseases and who are under professional supervision, particularly those with severe renal disease, should not make use of the information contained herein without the supervision of their attending physician.

All the recommendations and procedures herein contained are made without guarantee on the part of the author or the publisher, their agents, or employees. The author and publisher disclaim all liability in connection with the use of the information presented herein.

Persistent unintentional dehydration
in the human body can manifest
itself in as many ways as we in
modern medicine have identified as
"diseases of unknown etiology."

Preface

The National Library of Medicine in Bethesda, MD, held an exhibition on asthma in 1999. The mission statement of the exhibition and the historical progress of our present understanding of asthma are presented here to show that, although the disease has been around for thousands of years, its outcome has not changed. More people suffer from and die of asthma today than ever before. But the exhibition was designed to say that "we have made progress; we now have so many medications designed to help asthmatics." Nowhere was there any indication that the "system" is in search of understanding the cause and finding a natural cure for asthma. The focus is on asthma management. To show that something substantial is being done, research is said to focus on the discipline of genetics to pinpoint the disease!

Whereas the present structure of thought on asthma, as presented by the exhibition, is based on "traditional views," this book is designed to present a different perspective and approach to the understanding and natural prevention and cure of asthma. To highlight the difference between past thoughts and the future possibilities addressed in this book, some of the salient points of the exhibition are presented below. Let us begin with the mission statement of the exhibition.

"People everywhere in every age have struggled with asthma in different ways, but the feeling of breathlessness remains central to the disease. Today, asthma is a serious, widespread problem affecting an estimated 15 million in the United States. But what is asthma? Who has asthma and why? Have its prevalence and impact grown dramatically in our times? Can it be managed, prevented, or cured? How do people cope with asthma?

"To search for answers, this exhibit examines the medical and human history of asthma. The times and the places in which people live shape their experience of the disease. Healers battle it using the tools and knowledge of their time. People from all walks of life are here—poets and politicians, doctors and demagogues, singers and sports heroes—all who have responded valiantly, often creatively, to the challenges of living productively with asthma. The exhibition concludes with resources of coping with asthma today, and a glimpse of what the future might bring."

The exhibition then named a number of famous asthma sufferers, including composer, Ludwig von Beethoven; Russian Czar, Peter the Great; former U.S. presidents, Calvin Coolidge, Theodore Roosevelt and John F. Kennedy; and actors, Elizabeth Taylor, Liza Minnelli and Jason Alexander.

Some other information presented at the exhibition follows.

Asthma is a word of Greek origin. It means *gasping*. The Chinese understood that *"wheezy breathing"* was, like all other diseases, a symptom of imbalance in the life forces they called *Qi* or *Chi*. Physicians restored *Qi* by means of herbs, acupuncture, moxibustion (moxa is a plant that the Chinese burned on the skin for treatment of some diseases), massage, diet and exercise. The treatment directed to the whole person rather than focusing on a single organ or system.

"The Sanskrit word 'prana' means wind and soul as well as breath, and the connection of soul and breath hints at the close connection between mind, body and spirit in Hindu philosophy. Yoga developed by ancient Hindu philosophers as a spiritual discipline uses control of breathing to enhance meditation. Traditional Indian medicine taught patients these breathing techniques to use in managing their asthma.

"Native American peoples followed different healing practices combining spiritual remedies with herbal and other folk medicine. The Native American tribes were the first peoples to use tobacco (later very popular in Europe) as a remedy for asthma."

At the end of the nineteenth century, manufactured medications containing as primary ingredients alcohol, morphine and cocaine came into existence and were used freely. "Until the twentieth century, smoking cigarettes and pipes were the only ways of delivering medications directly into the bronchial tubes and the lungs. The cigarettes contained as asthma medication tobacco, or nitrate powders, plant-derived stramonium, or cubeb." (Cubeb is a small, spicy berry from Java and other East Indian islands.)

At the same time, experiments were being conducted on other methods of delivering medications into the lungs using air or steam instead of smoke. It is interesting to note that by the end of 1998, the pharmaceutical industry had succeeded in delivering medications into the lungs using air, and 38 different bronchiodilator drugs were marketed in the United States alone.

Even with all the claimed progress and ongoing research, more people suffer from asthma today than ever before. In the 20 years from 1975 to 1995, death from asthma among the Black community in the United States almost tripled from just under 1.5 per 100,000 deaths to over 4 per 100,000 deaths. Deaths from asthma among the Whites and Asians doubled in the same period.

The surge in asthma occurrence from 1980 to 1994 is testimony to the blatant inadequacies of the preventive approach to this problem.

- In the 14 years from 1980 to 1994, the number of asthma sufferers aged 0-4 years increased staggeringly from 2,000 to 6,000 per 100,000 population—a 300 percent increase!

- Among the age group of 5-14, the rate doubled from 3,500 to more than 7,000 per 100,000 population.

- The number among the age group of 15-34 doubled from 2,500 to 5,000 per 100,000 population.

- Among the age group of 35-64, the number increased from about 3,000 to 4,000 per 100,000 population.

- Among the age group of 65 and over, the number increased from 2,400 to 3,000—a 25 percent increase.

Asthma is becoming a serious concern in our society. In a Special Report on February 23, 1998, the *New York Daily News* claimed that 500,000 New Yorkers have asthma and called the disease "The Silent Killer."

The exhibition asked a number of questions and then tried to answer them in a way that suits the prevalent thinking.

"What is asthma? Four distinct, although overlapping, answers have endured in western medicine from the late nineteenth century to the present day—asthma as a primary disorder of the lungs, an allergic condition, a disease associated with environmental irritants, and a disease linked to emotional distress.

"Over time, asthma sufferers have sought relief from experts in lung disease, allergists, general practitioners, and psychiatrists. People's experiences with asthma have always been influenced by the kind of practitioners they consulted and the times and places in which they lived.

"Current scientific and clinical thinking integrates these four perspectives by emphasizing that asthma control requires a combination of medications, reducing environmental exposure, and improving patients' coping skill. And research now focuses on interactions of genetics, the environment and the immune system in causing asthma," the exhibition material stated. *The Washington Post Magazine*, October 31, 1999, asks a pertinent question of all those who claimed asthma is a genetic disease. "Asthma has a strong genetic component, but the gene pool hasn't changed in just two decades. What have we done to make it so hard for so many to breathe?"

From this page onward, we are going to apply Albert Einstein's famous quotation: *"The significant problems we have cannot be solved at the same level of thinking with which we created them,"* and present a new and more elevated scientific perspective to explain asthma. You, the reader, are invited to help eradicate this monument to present-day medical stupidity from the list of human diseases!

All that we need to do is to expunge commercial considerations from our subconscious minds and employ the motivating forces of empathy and sincerity for our scientific thoughts. After all, we need to be concerned for over 12 million constantly "suffocating" and death-threatened children. No parent should have to be in the position of watching his or her child battle to breathe when a simple, natural, and free cure for asthma is available. This book introduces you to that cure.

To silence the would-be critics, I have included in the book many, many testimonials, to the point that my copyeditors think there are too many of them. I do not consider them too many. Each one represents the story of long-awaited triumph over one condition from so many "killer-mistakes" in our, so-called, science-based medicine of the twentieth century.

In the chapter on lupus, I also explain why "lupus" is another label attached to a number of concurrently occurring complications of chronic unintentional dehydration.

F. Batmanghelidj, M.D.
March, 2000

1

Asthma No More

Water, water everywhere, not enough did we drink.
Water, water everywhere, still our lungs did shriek and shrink.

The greatest tragedy in medical history is the assumption or unspoken premise that "dry mouth" is the only sign of the body's water needs. The whole structure of modern medicine is built on this pitifully flawed and, for want of a stronger word, moronic assumption that brings about painful, premature death to so many millions of people. They suffer because they do not know they are only thirsty.

The human body uses a different logic to the basic "dry mouth" premise that is the cornerstone and very foundation of "modern medical science": to be able to chew and swallow, and to facilitate and lubricate this primary function, ample saliva is produced even if the rest of the body is short of water. In any case, water is too important to the body to only signal its shortage by experiencing a dry mouth. This mistake in medical thinking has given birth to the self-expanding "sick care system" that survives and thrives on people being sick.

It is now clinically and scientifically clear that the human body has many other distinct ways of showing its general or local water needs. Depending on where there is water shortage—

drought—many localized complications, such as asthma, are produced.

Before we get into the topic of this book—*asthma, allergy and lupus*—let us have a general discussion on the subject of dehydration and the many different ways the human body can manifest its internal drought.

Naturally, to understand asthma we need to become alert to the other early indicators of water shortages in different parts of the body. One thing must be made clear. In dehydration, 66 percent of the water loss is taken from inside the cells in the drought-stricken area, 26 percent is taken from the environment outside and around the cells, and only 8 percent is lost from the blood circulation.

Since the blood vessels are not rigid pipes but are made of soft and muscular tissues, they constrict and tighten on the empty space and correct for the 8 percent shortage. This is the reason why, with most of the symptom-producing states of regional drought, routine blood tests do not show any abnormality, yet the patient develops sufficiently severe discomfort to seek professional advice.

This is also the reason why, even after exhaustive, expensive, and bill-padding checkups in the nation's hospitals and brand-name clinics, and oftentimes a clean bill of health, some people have dropped dead soon after their release. Their blood tests did not reveal the underlying damages of dehydration in their vital organs. You see, by and large, the blood that is circulating is pretty well standardized by the liver. Function-reducing dehydration in an outlying area of the body—that might even be shut off by decreased circulation to the area—will not show itself in the routine blood tests that are presently used for evaluating health problems. Thus, most blood tests results are inconsequential.

To understand dehydration, we need to *recognize the vital functions of water and recognize dehydration by the missing functions of water in the symptom-producing areas of the body.* I have focused full time on this topic for the past 20 years and have developed an insight into the body's different markers of "persistent unintentional dehydration."

It is my researched opinion that the human body has three categories of indicators that should be considered as representatives or outcomes of dehydration in some parts of the body. They are: perceptive indicators, crisis calls of the body for water, and adaptive drought management and water rationing programs. These newly understood indicators of dehydration are distinct and recognizable, and all are preventable, before irreversible damage takes place.

The Perceptive Indicators of Drought in the Body

The brain itself is 85 percent water and is most sensitive to dehydration. It shows its water shortage by any of the following:

1) Feeling tired when it is not the result of strenuous work—in its extreme form, chronic fatigue syndrome. Syndrome means any three or more conditions that are routinely seen together. Symptoms are, by and large, telltale indicators of serious dehydration-produced problems the body is facing. This topic is further discussed in the section on lupus and the formula for energy generation by water is presented in that section.

2) Feeling flushed. When circulation to the brain increases to allow more water to get to the brain, the face also gets additional blood flow. The arteries in the face and the brain have a common feeder vessel because the face needs more circulation to allow its nerves to communicate with the brain.

3) Feeling irritable with least cause—anger without control.

4) Feeling anxious without a justified cause—anxiety neurosis, panic disorder, and agoraphobia.

5) Feeling dejected and inadequate (low libido).

6) Feeling depressed—in its extreme form, depression and suicidal tendencies.

7) Cravings for beverages, and even alcohol, hard drugs and cigarettes.

These are the perceptive indicators that dehydration is affecting some aspects of the functions of the brain itself. Thus, at its onset, shortage of water in the brain can cause the loss of certain functions and can result in the general and mental conditions described above.

The Crisis Calls of the Body for Water

Among the second group of crisis symptoms and signs of water needs of the body are the different localized chronic pains. They include the following:

1) Heartburn

2) Dyspepsia

3) Rheumatoid joint pain

4) Back pain

5) Migraine headaches

6) Leg pain on walking

7) Fibromyalgia—muscle and soft tissue pain, to the point of causing muscular dystrophy

8) Colitis pain and its associated constipation

9) Anginal pain—a sign of most advanced water shortage in the heart and lung axis

10) Early morning sickness of pregnancy, indicating thirst of the fetus and the mother

Bad breath is also an indication of water shortage in the body. It is produced by fermentation of food that has not been washed away from inside the stomach, or by gases that leave the intestine and work their way upward to leave via the mouth.

What these pains and symptoms mean is simple. When there is water shortage in a part of the body that is active and being used, the "toxic waste and acid buildup" produced as a result of tissue metabolism is not cleared away. Nerve endings register the environmental change of chemistry with the brain. By producing the above classic pains, the brain tries to let the _conscious mind_ know of the impending problems that will be caused by the local drought. If the drought continues, permanent tissue damage will ensue—such as colon cancer that is associated with long-term constipation and colitis pain.

The eventual acid burn and damage that will result from the "unwashed" excess acidity is why the body signals local drought by producing pain. It wants to limit activity to prevent more acid and toxic waste formation. This pain is similar to the whistle of a smoke detector, warning of a fire that might burn a house and its occupants. Pain is supposed to tell our conscious—but preoccupied and forgetful—minds that the acid buildup in the area will soon set the local cells "on fire" and cause acid burns. Pain is the "local resident genes' cries of anguish" before their impending death. Normally, it is water that washes the acid away and prevents its accumulation and damage to the area, in the same way that water extinguishes fires.

Until this stage of brain function, everything is within the normal range of body physiology. In short, pain not caused by infection or injury means water shortage in the area of pain registration. Pain is a crisis call of the body for the water that is needed to wash the toxic waste away from the drought-stricken area. The basic problem in the presently practiced form of "presumed to be science-based" medicine is the lack of knowledge about the significance and importance of pain as a thirst signal of the body.

When the body is calling for water, the medical profession has been duped into prescribing chemical poisons that painfully and prematurely kill people. The tragedy is that we in medicine have become accustomed to arrogantly thinking we are doing our patients good by continuously prescribing these expensive and slow-acting lethal poisons. The most common outcome of their use is further deterioration of body physiology because they give a false impression of "killing the pain," but they are not correcting what causes the pain: *dehydration*. In the case of injury, the area swells—swelling means more water is being brought to the site—and it is the additional water that causes the pain to diminish and even disappear after an injury.

The Drought Management Programs of the Body

The body possesses water rationing programs when it is in drought. The main drought management programs of the body that have been labeled as diseases are—

1) Asthma and allergies

2) Hypertension

3) Old-age diabetes

4) Constipation and its complication of pain in the lower intestines, colitis pain

5) Autoimmune diseases, including lupus

These conditions are major health problems produced by persistent water shortage of the human body. For more information on the other aspects of persistent water shortage in the body, you should read my book, *Your Body's Many Cries for Water,* or listen to my taped seminar, *Water: Rx for a Healthier Pain-Free Life.* You might also want to take a look at my videotape, *"Cure Pain and Prevent Cancer,"* to see how drought in the body is the primary cause of cancer.

Anginal pain could often be a component of asthma in older people. It means they have shortness of breath and also the characteristic heart pain that is now associated with asthmatics' reduced capacity for air exchange and difficulty in breathing. In other words, the automatically active heart is not receiving enough water to wash out the toxic byproducts that affect its efficiency to function at the same time that the body has activated a drought management program that affects the air flow.

Both the lungs and the heart muscle exhibit an inflammatory process that is produced by dehydration—to bring more microcirculation to the sites of dehydration. That is what an inflammatory process means—"added circulation to cope with the problem." Inflammation can be caused by bacteria, *chemicals*, or an injury. In pain-producing dehydration, it is the buildup of local toxic chemicals—molecular byproducts of metabolism—in the drought-stricken area that triggers the onset of pain.

In this book, we will only discuss asthma, allergies and lupus as three of the complications of not drinking water on a regular basis, or of ignorantly substituting manufactured beverages that do more harm than good in place of the water that the body should receive.

The section on lupus is added to this book because a number of concurrently occurring indicators of locked-in drought management programs have been lumped together and labeled as an autoimmune disease, implying an autoallergy of the body to its own tissues. This categorization of a number of symptoms and complications of prolonged drought in the body as an autoimmune disease commands a hearing in this book, in addition to asthma and allergies.

In Chapter 10, *Asthma Eradication: It's History in the Making,* you will learn the extent of the effort I have made to get the "administration" to engage itself in the research and spread of my discovery that asthma is caused by water and salt deficiency in the body.

Had "they" taken up this line of research when I pleaded with them, writing this book would have been unnecessary. Alas, they ignored my call and the public's interest, forcing me to write the pages that follow and placing a demand on you to become educated about the many ways your body talks to you.

2

Asthma and Allergies

The Breathing Process

To understand asthma, one needs to have some idea of the anatomy of the lungs and chest. Figures 1 to 7 explain the mechanical aspects of breathing. Further on, I will explain how the volume of the air we need to breathe becomes affected if there is not enough water in the body.

On average, we breathe about 12 times a minute and exchange 500 ccs of air each time. The average air exchange in normal breathing is about 6,000 ccs of air a minute. People who become short of breath can breathe up to 50 times a minute and draw in about 3,000 to 4,000 ccs at a time—if their air passageways are open. They cannot sustain this rate of air flow for very long. The physiology of expiration will not keep up and the volume of air exchanged will decrease drastically.

The nasal passageways perform three very important functions. The folds on the middle wall between the two passages divide the air current into three streams on each side that is in close contact with the moist mucosa. The air becomes moist. It is warmed to a comfortable temperature and filtered from its suspended particles that stick to the moist surface of the nasal mucosa.

CHEST EXPANSION CREATES VACUUM AND DRAWS AIR INTO THE LUNGS

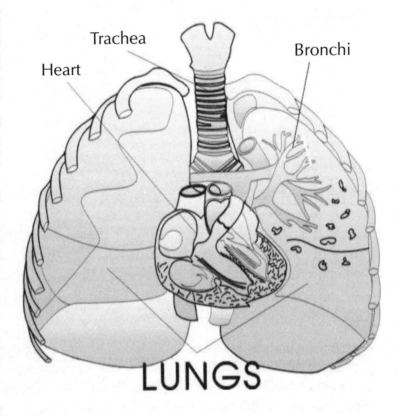

Figure 1. The chest cavity contains five lung segments or lobes. The two left lobes fill the left side of the chest cavity. The three right lobes, the upper, middle, and lower lobes, fill the right chest cavity. The lungs are separated from the chest wall by a thin, silky membrane covering—pleura—that allows the lungs to expand and contract without sticking to the chest wall. The heart is cradled between the right and the left lungs—more to the left side.

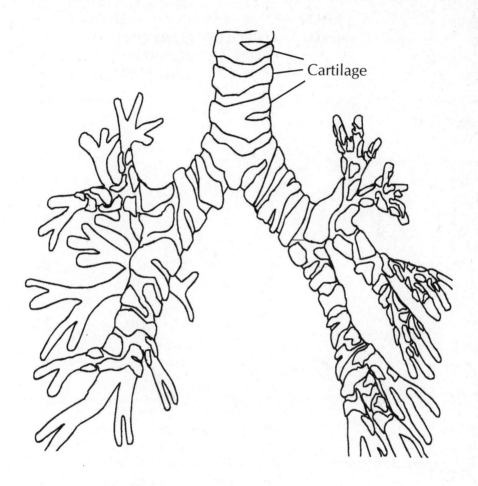

Cartilage

Figure 2. The inverted bronchial tree, with its smaller branches—bronchioles—spanning downward and outward, acts as the scaffolding for the myriad air sacs that are the site of gas exchange in the lungs. Starting from the top, interrupted rings of cartilage give the bronchial tree its firm, tube-like structure and form at the same time that it is supple. In its lower extremities, the bronchioles are made of rings of soft muscular and fibrous tissue and no cartilage. In children, the air pipes are smaller and their cartilage is less formed and firm. This is why children are more susceptible to tighter closing of their air passageways.

BRONCHIOLES

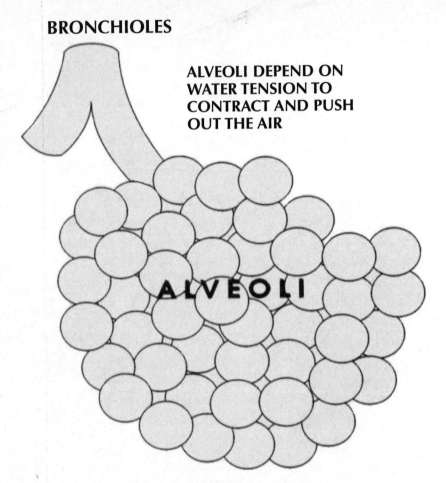

ALVEOLI DEPEND ON WATER TENSION TO CONTRACT AND PUSH OUT THE AIR

ALVEOLI

Figure 3. Attached to the bronchioles are the air sacs, or alveoli. They are much like bunches of grapes attached to the stem by their stalks, except that the "stem and stalks" in the lungs are air tubes through which air flows in and out of the alveoli. In asthma, it is the bronchioles that constrict and block the flow of air upward and outward. The air sacs remain overinflated. When you think of your lungs, think of bunches of grapes, except the "berries" of the lungs are full of air, not juice. If their "skin" were to be dehydrated, they would break down and collapse into one another and lose function. That is why, in dehydration, the air sacs are inflated and "sealed off" from the outside air to enable them to keep their shape and maintain their humidity. Only if well hydrated are all the air sacs opened up for air exchange.

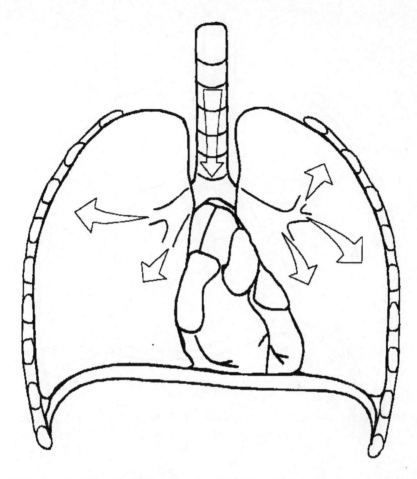

Figure 4. The chest cavity is sealed at its base and separated from the abdominal content by a muscular dome—the diaphragm. When the dome contracts, it flattens and pulls the lower ribs down with it. At the same time, it pushes the abdominal content downward, creating more space in the chest cavity. Air is sucked into the lungs because of the vacuum that is created. This is how we inhale air into the lungs.

When we only rely on the diaphragm for drawing air into the lungs, the process is called abdominal breathing. Abdominal breathing is a shallow form of breathing and the lungs are not fully aerated. The abdominal muscles also help in this form of breathing by relaxing when the diaphragm pushes the abdominal content downward.

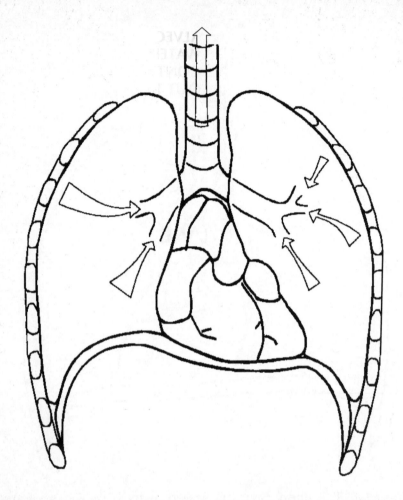

Figure 5. When gases have been exchanged and the air in the
lungs must be pushed out, the diaphragm relaxes and achieves its
dome-like form. The lower ribs go back to their resting position
and the "<u>elastic recoil of the lungs</u>" exerts a form of squeeze on
the lungs full of air. The air is pushed out until the act of exhala-
tion is complete. The amount of air normally exchanged in quiet
breathing is about 500 cubic centimeters (ccs) of the lungs' total
capacity of about 5,500 ccs.

Deep breathing involves the active expansion and contraction
of the chest wall itself. The ribs are pulled up to expand the cavity inside the chest. In very deep breathing, the volume of air
exchange is about 3,000 to 3,500 ccs.

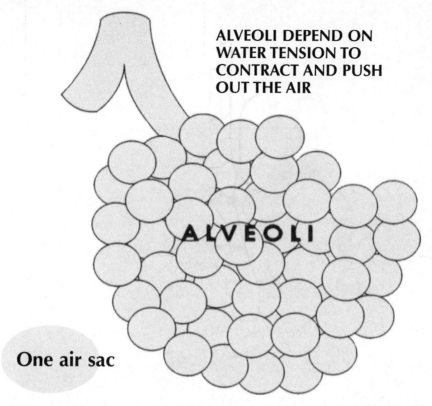

ALVEOLI DEPEND ON
WATER TENSION TO
CONTRACT AND PUSH
OUT THE AIR

ALVEOLI

One air sac

Figure 6. The movement of the chest wall and the diaphragm is not enough to <u>uniformly</u> push the air out of the alveoli—air sacs—throughout the lungs. There are a myriad air sacs in the lungs. Each one needs to expel the air that it has received during the act of inhalation. Here is the secret. As we inhale, the same vacuum that draws in air also draws tiny molecules of water into all of the air sacs. Beads of water have the natural property of being attracted to each other. They join together and form larger clumps of water that cover the inside wall of the air sacs.

The force that pulls molecules of water together is called the *"surface tension of water."* This force also acts on the wall of the air sacs and forces them to shrink as the water molecules clump together. The force created by the surface tension of water inside the air sacs adds to the force brought to bear by *recoil contraction* of the lung tissue itself, and makes the air sacs contract uniformly throughout the lungs and push out some of the air that is inside them.

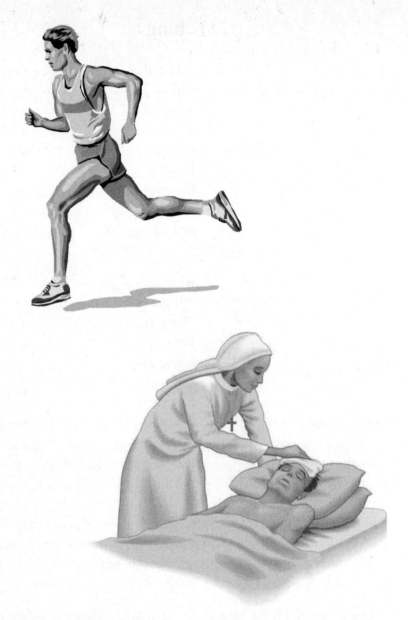

Figure 7. Athletes during severe exertion and very sick people fighting for survival demonstrate drastic demands on their breathing process, such as heavy breathing or heaving expansion and contraction of the chest. The sick with this kind of breathing problem are nowadays nursed in an oxygen tent or with forced oxygen delivered through a nasal tube to reduce their struggle for oxygen supply. Young athletes have the greatest lung capacity.

Coughing

Coughing seen in some with breathing problems involves a rapid drawing of about two liters of air into the lungs followed by tight closing of the vocal chords and the air valve (epiglottis) on the trachea above the "voice box." At the same time, the abdominal muscles and muscles connecting the ribs together contract forcefully and put the air in the lungs under great pressure. All of a sudden, the vocal chords and the epiglottis open widely, the air in the lungs bursts out, and any loose particle in the pathway becomes a projectile with a speed of about 75 to 100 miles an hour.

Coughing is part of the cleansing mechanism for the lung tissue that is in constant contact with particles suspended in the air that enters through the nose. In lung infections and irritation of the air pipes (the bronchus and bronchioles), the cough reflex is triggered and a person can cough to exhaustion. This type of a cough is normally dry and can become bothersome. Asthmatics usually develop such a dry cough before their shortness of breath and gasping for air become obvious. *It is this initial cough that should be recognized as a primary indicator of an impending asthma attack.* The cough seems to be caused by the same process that will stimulate the secretion of mucus for plugging the bronchioles.

"The significant problems we have
cannot be solved at the same level
of thinking with which we created
them." — **Albert Einstein**

3

Asthmatics and Their Acid/Alkali Balance

What is the ideal acid/alkali (pH) balance and how is it achieved? A pH of 7.4 inside the cells and 7.3 to 7.2 in the blood is an ideal reading. These numbers are the readings on a scale designed to measure the degree of acidity in the body. From 1 to 7 is the acid range of pH, with 1 being more acid than 7. From 7 to 14 on the scale is the alkaline range of pH, with 7 being less alkaline than 14. On the pH scale, 7 is neutral. Thus, the health-ensuring functions of the body in its internal and external cellular environment must remain within the above-mentioned *exact range.*

If the blood begins to become acidic, the body starts producing drastic symptoms. According to Guyton's *Textbook of Medical Physiology,* 8th Edition, page 331, *"The lower limit at which a person can live more than a few hours is about 6.8 and the upper limit approximately 8.0."* In other words, if the pH of blood reached about 6.8, and stayed at that level for a few hours, a person could only live for a few hours. Similarly, a drastic shift toward an alkaline range—a blood pH of 8 for a few hours— would be life-threatening. People who advertise and sell pH-altering filters and tell their customers to drink strong alkaline water should be cautious with their statements and advice. They can very easily hurt their unsuspecting customers. Consumers who have such filters should not drink alkaline water constantly.

The body has many acid-buffering mechanisms that regulate the acid/alkali balance of its inner environment. *One major mechanism is attached to the breathing process.*

The gas exchanges in the lungs regulate the acidity of the body. Hemoglobin is a very complex molecule that delivers carbon dioxide to the lung tissue to be released into the air that is about to leave the body and collects oxygen to circulate throughout the body. Each hemoglobin molecule is made up of four iron-containing units attached to one another, similar to the Figure 8 on the right. Each red cell contains a certain amount of these hemoglobin molecules—depending on the efficiency of the blood-forming mechanisms.

As the hemoglobin unit rotates on its axis, it releases the carbon dioxide it collected from the outlying parts of the body into the water environment inside the red cell and in its place picks up four oxygen molecules that enter the red cell. As the freed carbon dioxide concentration inside the red cells increases, it escapes into the air in the air sacs. *When carbon dioxide leaves the lungs, the body fluids become more alkaline*—an ideal situation for a healthy body.

Figure 8

Hemoglobin does something else that is very important. It collects excess hydrogen atoms—a very strong acid factor—and attaches them to its own protein structure and neutralizes their damage-causing acidity. In asthma attacks, the escape of excess hydrogen atoms in the low volume exhaled air can make it acidic. Thus, breathing normally is vital for the acid/alkali balance of the body—by far the most important pH-regulating mechanism the body possesses. The direct relationship of air exchange in the lungs and effective pH regulation is the reason deep breathing is encouraged in all exercise protocols and in yoga.

In asthmatics, because of the low rate of air exchange in their lungs, this acid-eliminating mechanism is inefficient and is the main source of danger to their lives. Every year, many thousands of asthmatics die from this imbalance of their body physiology. The actual "death punch" takes place in the brain that swells from inefficient oxygen supply and faulty pH regulation that causes the brain cell environment to become fatally acidic.

By now, you have some indication of the importance of water to the act of breathing and forcing the air out of our lungs. You should also know that water is vital for enabling the red blood cells to pick up more oxygen as they pass through the lungs. Water is also very important in acid/alkali regulation by the kidneys: when the kidneys form more urine, they get rid of the excess hydrogen ions that would otherwise acid-burn some important parts inside the cells that produce the extra hydrogen.

Salt is also vital for the regulation of the acid/alkali balance in the body, particularly for the brain cells. The element sodium in salt is involved in the extraction of acid radicals from inside the cells for secretion by the kidneys. Sodium is also involved in the formation of bicarbonate soda in the mucus layer of the stomach that protects its cell lining from the acid inside the stomach cavity. Sodium bicarbonate is also produced by the pancreas and secreted into the first part of the intestine at the same moment that the acid content of the stomach enters the intestine.

Believe it or not, low sodium (salt) in the diet can affect all of these functions. Asthmatics are particularly cautioned about the detrimental effects of a low-salt diet. In my opinion, asthma occurs by and large as the compounding effect of low salt intake on top of an establishing dehydration in the body.

"A new scientific truth is not usually
presented in a way to convince its
opponents. Rather, they die off, and
a rising generation is familiarized
with the truth from the start."

Max Planck

4

Questions and Answers About Asthma and Allergies

When talking about the simplicity of the curative role of water in my physiologic approach to the treatment of asthma and allergies, I am faced with the types of questions listed below. For the benefit of some 17 million asthmatic children and adults, and 50 million suffering from allergies, the following explanations should help them understand why water is the best natural medication for the prevention and treatment of these conditions.

Question: Why has my doctor never told me about this water cure for asthma?

Answer: As you can see, even we in the medical profession need to learn more about the medicinal properties of water and its importance to our health. You see, water, from which all life emerged, is the unifying factor that gives life to life. Doctors recommend "fluids" intake and assume that any fluid you take will act like water. This is what we have all been taught at school. We are not well informed about the intricate functions of water in the human body. Furthermore, we are not decisive in our instruction to "take fluids" and how much! We do not yet understand chronic unintentional dehydration. We do not yet understand that the final effect of some of the "designer drinks" we take is not necessarily as healthful for the body as the simple water that it needs.

Water is the very basic element that interconnects the normal functions of all structures that go to make our body into a single unit of "water-dependent" life on land. Water is the "cash flow" of the body. However, although there is plenty of water for our drinking needs, and we all know it is good for us, the human body can still become chronically dehydrated. We don't know or understand what happens to our bodies if we do not drink water on a regular basis. We, therefore, give lip service to the importance of water, but shortchange our bodies all the time!

Furthermore, all the fluids that contain caffeine and alcohol dehydrate us and cannot replace the water needs of the human body. Caffeine and alcohol force the kidneys to flush some of the water reserves of the body. More water will leave the body than is contained in the drink. Hot drinks and alcohol also open the skin pores and increase water loss from the surface area of the body. We also lose some salt, the element that retains water in the body.

Question: Then all I have to do is to make sure I drink plenty of water when I feel thirsty. Right?

Answer: Wrong. As I have already explained, "dry mouth" is not an accurate sign of water shortage in our bodies. There is an overriding mechanism that sees to it that we manufacture ample saliva through our salivary glands, even when we are comparatively dehydrated. The reason for this is twofold: one, to be able to lubricate the foods we eat during chewing and swallowing; two, to make available to the stomach for the process of digestion of food some watery, alkaline saliva when not enough water in the body is taken by mouth to be resecreted directly into the stomach to facilitate the breakdown of food. Normally when we drink a glass of water, it gets into the intestines and, within a half hour, is resecreted into the stomach to prepare that organ to receive food. Thus, dehydration of the body that can very silently cause damage will not necessarily cause a dry mouth.

The misconception about "dry mouth" as an accurate indicator of body water shortage has steered medical research off course for the last 100 years. At the turn of the century, Walter Bradford Cannon, an English physician, forced the broad acceptance of his very limited view that a "dry mouth state" is the only sign of thirst in the human body. A few years earlier, Maurice Shiff, a French scientist, had said that thirst in the body produces a more generalized feeling. Alas, the French view did not prevail. If the medical community had studied Mr. Shiff's opinion about the other indicators of body dehydration at that time, we would have been 100 years ahead of the game that is only now being understood.

Even at the very end of the twentieth century, it is not generally known at what stage the human body is thirsty and becoming dehydrated. It is not fully appreciated what devastating damage is caused by a slowly establishing unintentional dehydration in our bodies, just because we do not recognize our bodies' ways of showing true thirst! We need to realize we have to prevent dehydration and not wait for it to show itself. We need to realize that dehydration may not necessarily be generalized, that some special rationing priorities become established. Priorities for the distribution of the available water *do exist,* and a *very ruthless* water distribution program becomes automatically operational— hence, in some, asthma to the point of death!!

My clinical experience and scientific research tell me that the human body possesses a number of different, highly sophisticated, emergency thirst signals. We need to be aware of these newly discovered indicators of water shortage in our body. Water as a natural medicine is free; all you might need to do to cure some of your health problems could be a slight modification in your daily choice of "fluids" intake. You assume all "fluids" are as good as water for the human body. As I explained, just because there is water in some drinks, it does not necessarily follow that these drinks work in the same way as simple water.

Question: What has all this got to do with asthma?

Answer: Asthma and allergy—conditions mainly treated with different kinds of antihistamine medications—are important indicators of dehydration in the body. Histamine is a most important neurotransmitter that primarily regulates the thirst mechanism for increased water intake. It also establishes a system for rationing the available water in the body during dehydration. Histamine is a most noble element employed in the drought management of our bodies. It is with us from the first moments of life in the uterus. It is the *"wet-nurse"* to the single-cell fetus. It facilitates the flow of water and nutrients to the fertilized ovum and helps it divide into two daughter cells. It then facilitates the division of the new cells for the duration of pregnancy until a fully developed child is born nine months later. Histamine is a growth factor in the body. This is why growing children produce more histamine in their bodies.

Histamine is not the villain that we have been led to believe. The way the chemical industry has dictated its view of histamine in our treatment protocols shows malice on the industry's part and exposes the medical profession's ignorance of the human body. We in medical practice have traditionally concentrated on detailed research of the "solids" composition of the body and have ignored the role of water that dissolves these solids. That is why we have never understood the symptoms and signs of chronic drought in the human body!

In dehydration, histamine production and its activity increase greatly. In this phase of its activity, histamine also generates the emergency thirst signals and indicators of its water rationing program that is in operation. Increased histamine release in the lungs causes the spasm of the bronchioles.

This natural spasmodic action of histamine on the bronchial tubes is part of the design of the body to conserve water that would normally evaporate during breathing. The winter steam or fog that you see when you breathe out in cold weather is water that is leaving your lungs as you breathe.

We breathe approximately 720 times an hour. Imagine how much water we lose through breathing in one hour, in one day, in one week! Could we live for long if we did not replace the water loss from our lungs? When we neglect to replace this water loss, how does the body deal with this crisis? Initially, and stage by stage, the drought management programs of the body are activated. In some, bronchial constriction—asthma—is the first reaction to dehydration. Children are more susceptible to asthma than adults. Their bodies are growing all the time and every cell in an expanding body needs 75 percent of its volume in water. At the same time, children's bronchial trees are smaller and less rigid, and can be constricted more efficiently than fully developed bronchial trees with firm cartilage support in their structure. Children's bodies also have less of a water reserve to tap into for redistribution. These are the reasons children exhibit shortness of breath—asthma—more readily than adults when they become dehydrated.

Attacks of asthma during exercise and stress are also part of the water preservation and crisis management process during dehydration. An asthma attack after eating is a classic indicator of dehydration. If we eat food and don't drink water, in order to digest and "liquefy" the food we have stuffed into the stomach, the water that is needed to complete the digestion process is borrowed from the rest of the body. This repeated scrounging of water from here and there in an already "drought-stricken" person predisposed to asthma will precipitate an asthma attack.

Both emotional and physical stress cause more acute dehydration in an already dehydrated body. The "free" water that is available for new functions is utilized very rapidly in the chemical reactions needed to cope with any particular form of stress, or for opening the vascular bed in the muscles during physical activity. This is why asthmatics are naturally fearful of food and exercise.

Question: I am still not too clear on what histamine does. Can you explain further?

Answer: When we become dehydrated, histamine sees to it that the available water in the body is strictly preserved and is distributed according to a priority of function. With increased water supply to the body, histamine production and its excess release are inhibited proportionately.

The effect of dehydration and subsequent hydration on the rate of histamine production within the cells that produce it— mast cells that are resident in all tissues, and basophil white cells that circulate with the rest of the white cells in blood circulation—has been demonstrated in several animal experiments. Dehydration causes these special histamine-producing cells to manufacture more of the chemical. Once fully hydrated, these cells decrease their rate of histamine manufacture and release. It is now physiologically apparent that water by itself has very strong, natural antihistaminic properties in the bodies of most living species, mankind included. Scientists have been aware of this fact for many years, but the medical profession is still in the dark; hence our present health care crisis and its costs.

Histamine also silently regulates most important aspects of the immune system of the body. All the white cells of the body have on their membranes one or other of the two types of receiving points that are known for this neurotransmitter. These receiving points, called receptors, are highly specific for their impact on the interior of the cells that have them.

However, with increased activity for histamine's water regulatory responsibilities, some of histamine's immune system regulatory activities become inhibited to accommodate its immediately more vital drought management programs. The reason for the development of this inhibitory mechanism is simple. It is designed in a way that, if there is dehydration and more histamine is produced for its drought management program, this increased rate of histamine production will not "heat up" the activity of the immune system in the same way that would be done if there was an infection. This process is the reason why when you have an infection, it is prudent to drink lots of *water.*

Question: How exactly does excess histamine depress the immune system and cause allergies?

Answer: There are a great number of special white cells in the bone marrow that are sensitive to histamine. Some of these resident white cells in the bone marrow have an inhibitory action and some have a stimulating action on the activity of the mother cells in the bone marrow that manufacture all the cells that are seen within the circulating blood. There are twice as many of these inhibitory white cells located in the bone marrow as there are cells that stimulate the immune system. Thus, dehydration that causes the production and release of more than a certain amount of histamine will, in the long run, automatically suppress the immune system of the body—at its bone marrow site. This is exactly how and why the immune system cannot cope in other diseases, including cancer, when the body has suffered "drought" for some time.

However, even if the immune system is suppressed, since there is more than the normal rate of histamine production and its storage because of prolonged dehydration, a stimulus for the release of histamine from its immune system side of activity will produce a greater quantity of histamine release into the tissues. At the same time, antibody production will be proportionately inhibited. In dehydration, the immune system cannot effectively cope with all the antigens that flood the airways and the exposed membranes of the eyes that also need to be constantly kept moist.

Dehydration would normally produce dry membranes in the nose and eyes were it not for the action of histamine and its subordinate chemicals that allocate an increased distribution of water to these organs. In the eyes, the tear-producing glands must now produce more secretion, not only to keep the eyes moist, but also to wash the offending pollen away from the delicate membranes of the eyelids and eyeballs. Histamine's initiation of activity for the secretion of water onto the delicate membranes covering the eyes and the nasal passageways must naturally be exaggerated.

The tear and nasal secretions have to be copious, and the watery secretions must also wash and cleanse the exposed membranes. This is the only way the body defends itself against different varieties of *offending pollens that are not neutralized by the appropriate antibodies that are less available in dehydration.* In other words, the alternative way of dealing with offending pollen in dehydration is to wash it away—that is why we develop the discomfort of watery eyes and nose. Allergy to pollen occurs as a result of chronic dehydration in the human body. Otherwise, the norm would be that everyone would suffer from allergy! Allergic reactions to foods obey the same principle. The more "solid" the foods we eat—breakdown, digestion and absorption of solid food needs lots of water—the more allergic reactions can ensue if one is dehydrated.

Remember, not everyone is allergic. It is the norm not to be allergic. It is the norm to be well hydrated. It is only as a result of the successful push of the beverage industry that we tend to substitute pleasant-tasting but less-than-healthful drinks in place of natural water that the body is designed to receive.

Question: Do you mean to say one can prevent asthma and allergy by drinking more water?

Answer: Yes, you can do it naturally. When you understand the physiology of the human body and the role of histamine in its water regulation and drought management, you realize that chronic dehydration, in a vast majority of people, is the primary cause of allergies and asthma. Increased water intake—on a forced, regular basis—should be adopted as a preventive measure as well as the treatment of choice. In those who have had attacks of asthma or allergic reactions to different pollens or foods, more strict attention to daily water intake should become a preemptive measure. These people will also have other indicators of dehydration that they need to recognize and treat accordingly before a crisis attack of asthma endangers their lives and exposes them to possible premature death. Don't forget, the chemical pathways dealing with dehydration have no "brain"; they rush forward like a cascade. They are actually called "chemical cascades." These dehydration-induced chemical cascades kill many thousands of asthmatics a year. They are easily "turned off" by water and salt, two strong, natural antihistamines.

Certain chemicals and toxic gases may also precipitate an episode of shortness of breath or irritable coughs that herald an impending asthma attack. The lungs are shut down to prevent a toxic chemical gaining access to the interior of the body and injuring its delicate cells, particularly the brain cells.

To stress the importance of being alert to chemical sensitivity, let me tell you about myself. My body is very reactive to certain chemicals. For years, I used creams or sprays against mosquitoes when I traveled to areas where there were malaria-carrying mosquitoes. I noticed that some of these creams and sprays made my skin red and swollen. I stopped using them and was careful not to expose myself to the mosquitoes.

As a young man studying at St. Mary's Hospital Medical School, and subsequently as a doctor working there, I became aware of a mild allergic reaction to what I thought was chemicals with which I must have come into contact. I did not pay much attention since the reactions did not appear to be serious. I also became sensitive to my leather watchband. When I exercised and the watchband became wet with perspiration, the skin under the band would become red, itchy and swollen. I had to wear metal watchbands. The same skin reaction occurred in the area under my hip pocket where I carried my leather wallet. It seems the sweat dissolved the chemicals used to cure the leather, and these chemicals would make contact with the skin and cause the inflammation or *contact dermatitis*.

Bear with me through my story of chemical sensitivity, as I want to introduce you to an important but, until now, not-thought-of trigger mechanism for asthma attacks.

In the early 60s, the first antibiotic against fungal infections was introduced onto the market. It was related to penicillin. The drug attached itself to the keratin layer of the skin, making it resistant to being penetrated by the fungus. I tested it against a type of nail fungus that was eating into the tips of two fingers of a five-year-old girl. It worked wonders and prevented the spread of the fungus to her other fingers. The infection cleared in a few days.

Some time later, I developed a fungal infection between my toes. I played many hours of tennis each day, and the sweat and humidity must have provided the ideal environment for the kinds of fungi that are prevalent in shower rooms. I tried to get rid of the infection with my newly found antibiotic. In about two weeks, I became allergic to the drug and my immune system reacted to the new kertain-antibiotic combination. I began to lose the hair on my legs, arms, trunk, shoulders, and back of my neck. I managed to save some hair on my head by immediately starting cortisone treatment.

Many years later, I was swimming one late summer afternoon in New Jersey when I noticed I was being eaten up by the "ladies of the night." Rather than abandoning the pleasure of my swim, I reached for a can of mosquito repellent that my sister-in-law had in her bag and sprayed my neck and shoulders. Instantly I realized the folly of this thoughtless action. My lips began to swell and become numb. Within a few minutes we reached the emergency department of Princeton Medical Center. I asked the nurse to give me an injection of adrenaline first and fill out the forms afterwards. She took a look at my face and rushed me to the emergency room where the resident doctor rushed to my side and told the nurse to give me an injection to arrest the progress of my allergic reaction.

By now you know that I also acquire medical knowledge from my body's reactions to certain situations, and I am alert to its capability of remembering and recognizing the elements that are not good for it. The same processes involved in the recognition of toxic chemicals are available in all of us. We need to become alert to this phenomenon. Each of us has to become a detective if we are to live healthily in our present commerce-driven society where we are pushed more and more to use chemical products that are deemed "good" for our bodies.

As you will see in the story that follows, I recently became a victim again of chemicals used in a heavily advertised product. The story illustrates the seriousness of acquired allergy to chemicals.

I am a fairly healthy person. I walk and exercise, not as much as I should, but whenever I can get away from my work. I play golf. I walk the course and carry my own clubs. When I finish, I am almost as fresh as when I started. I do not experience shortness of breath. Often, when I cannot go out, I exercise on a stationary bicycle for 30 to 90 minutes. I get drenched with sweat but do not get short of breath.

Last fall in Florida, one night I suddenly felt short of breath and experienced a typical asthma attack when I was in bed. I was puzzled and concerned. Fortunately I had water and salt at my bedside. I drank two glasses of water and put a few grains of sea salt on my tongue. The shortness of breath decreased quickly and disappeared within a couple of minutes. The incident passed and I soon forgot about it.

A few nights later, however, I again had the same problem. I became very concerned and did not know why I was experiencing such a perplexing problem.

My wife is Chinese. She is intelligent and reads a lot. When she gets into a magazine she can easily read for a few hours without even shifting position! She is interested in reading new ideas and views. She has bought into the Western values of keeping healthy and maintaining her looks. She has accepted the idea that to retain one's youthful looks one does not use soap and water to clean one's face, but rather various creams to keep the skin moist.

I never suspected that anything in her cosmetic materials had become the arrow of my misfortune until she mentioned that she had discovered a new line of products that seemed to be effective and much cheaper than what she had been using previously. She was even very excited by the fact that a company known for its nonallergenic soaps had produced this line of products.

All of a sudden my attention was focused on when she had begun to use these new products. I started to do some detective work and discovered that she used a heavy dose of the night cream last thing at night before getting into bed. She showed me the products and I saw the night cream contained a cleansing solvent chemical designed to remove "whatever clogs the pores." It became clear to me that my body was reacting to whatever was in the night cream. The disclaimer and warning notice on the cream jar acknowledged the possibility of problems by instructing the user to discontinue its use at the slightest indication of a reaction.

I had a strong feeling that this new cleansing cream that was introduced into my breathing environment when I was close to my wife was the offending agent to which I was reacting. My body did not like what it was doing to my lung tissue and was telling me to keep away from it, even though that meant keeping away from my wife's face! I asked my wife not to use the cream again.

She did not buy into my request and explanations, and voiced her disbelief. After all, she had paid a lot of money to buy a few months' supply of the cream. She thought if she was discreet and used less of it on her face it would be harmless and I would not object. However, I still began to cough and became short of breath and had an asthma attack the next time I was close to her face when she had used the cleansing cream. My wife then realized that if a chemical agent was so hazardous to my health, then she too would be vulnerable. She stopped using that line of cosmetics and is now using "all-natural" products that contain no chemicals. Let us hope she does not buy into another advertising onslaught!

The moral of this story is twofold: one, be careful with beauty products that have too many ingredients, with most being chemicals; two, become curious about the chemical products you use routinely and for long periods of time. Your body will, sooner or later, react to the chemicals used in beauty products or sprays.

Naturally, chemicals that produce allergies are different from natural vegetable products, such as pollen, that the body has learned to neutralize by its array of antibodies that grip onto the offending "protein" and cover its chemically active "surface." Water helps in the adequate production and effectiveness of the body's natural antibodies that neutralize antigens at the location of their entry into the body, such as through the eyes, nose, lungs, and so on.

A well-hydrated body will produce more than enough "anti-body soldiers" to man the battlefield against offending intruders in the body, including dust mites and tiny organisms that can gain access to the interior of the body. The body's reaction to offending chemicals is different to its reaction against biological agents that possess proteins in their composition.

The body can mount a "foreign protein-specific antibody" defense system, but cannot protect itself against noxious gases and chemicals. This is why I became vulnerable to the chemical solvent but am not allergic to pollen or dust mites. My body produces antibodies to deal with these particles but has to shut down my lungs to prevent toxic gases or chemicals from gaining entry to my system. For your information, the liver is the organ that deals with chemical toxins and neutralizes them at a slow rate.

Question: How can you say water and salt cure asthma and allergies when they are said to be genetically determined disorders?

Answer: More and more research is directed at genetic aspects of disease. But what are they really saying when they say diseases are a genetically unavoidable outcome of living? What they want you to accept is that it is your own genetic "fault" if you have a health problem, and the best you can expect is that it can be controlled by your taking a commerce-driven treatment protocol.

I think this approach is a cop-out and is a result of many years of misdirected research into the cause of human diseases. Firstly, the genetic makeup of mankind has not changed so dramatically and rapidly over the years as to warrant such a dramatic rise in the occurance of various diseases. Cancer has been on the rise for the past 30 years, asthma has increased dramatically in the past 20 years, allergies, lupus, you name it, are occurring much more frequently than they were 50 years ago.

Does this mean the genetic pool has become so disease prone in such a short time? No! It means that the primary factor in disease production is not the genetic pool, but the lifestyle that people pursue that drastically shortens each phase of the ongoing transition from childhood to old age and death.

Question: How much water should one drink?

Answer: If you suffer from allergies and asthma, you should begin drinking water daily on a regular basis, and take salt regularly too—for more information, see the section on diet and salt. You should stop taking caffeine and alcohol in your drinks, at least until your condition has become normal. Always remember that some fluids may not be a suitable replacement for simple water, particularly for children (see the section on diet). People with normal heart and kidney function should begin drinking two glasses of water a half hour before each meal, and one glass of water two and a half hours after the meal. *Drink water any time you feel thirst, even in the middle of a meal.* Children need water for cell growth. Seventy-five percent of the cell volume during growth has to be filled with water. Naturally, smaller children need less water than grown-ups. A rough rule of thumb of how much water a person needs a day is half one's body weight in ounces of water. A 60-pound child then will need about 30 oz of water. Some children might need 3/4 of their body weight in ounces of water. They will also need to take some extra salt.

As we age, we lose our thirst sensation and do not recognize that our bodies are thirsty. Chronic dehydration in the elderly can cause heart and kidney damage. Those with heart problems and kidney disease, and who are under treatment, should increase their water intake slowly and, if possible, under the supervision of their physician. Urine production should increase with additional water intake. If, within two full days, there is no indication of more urine being produced, a physician should be consulted. The color of urine in a dehydrated person (who is not taking vitamins that could color the urine) is dark yellow to orange. In a better-hydrated person, the urine is lighter in color.

Children and adults who get asthma attacks with exercise and strenuous effort should always remember to drink water before they begin exercising and to stop drinking caffeine-containing sodas. *They should also take some salt before exercise*—salt will increase stamina during exercise. They should reduce their orange juice intake (if more than two glasses). Because of its high potassium content, orange juice in large quantities can predispose to attacks of asthma. The water needs of the body cannot be fully replaced by juices or other potassium-containing beverages. The same applies to too much milk. *It is safer to add a little salt to the orange juice to balance the sodium potassium intake when one wants to drink orange juice.*

Question: How can I use water to control or treat extensive allergic reactions?

Answer: For extensive allergic reactions, one should immediately drink at least three or four glasses of water and take a little salt to prevent circulation problems that can occur when circulation to the skin increases to the point of producing skin eruptions, blotchiness, and even edema or swelling. In this situation, water and salt will act as very strong antihistamines and will increase urine production so that the toxic material that has caused the eruptions can be flushed out with the urine.

At the same time, exposing the skin to water from the outside, such as by showering or bathing, will help to alleviate the itchiness and other symptoms. The best way to deal with this situation is to stand under a shower and change the water from hot to cold every minute. The water should be as hot and as cold as you can bear. By doing this, you will exhaust the chemical reserves of the local nerves and ultimately you will abort the reactive response of the nerve endings on the skin. Normally, five to ten minutes of hot and cold showers, ending with a cold shower, will take away itchiness completely.

Let me tell you about a case I treated in this way. A young man, 24 years old, had become allergic to something in his food and had developed a rash that covered him from the top of his head to almost his toes. He had an uncontrollable itch and desire to scratch, which had caused skin damage. He responded to this hot and cold method of treatment within minutes and his skin irritation ceased to bother him.

Using water on the outside of the body has medicinal values in many conditions. For example, if you are starting a cold, this treatment works well and is used in Scandinavian countries all the time. Basically, this is the logic behind saunas that are so popular in Scandinavia. People sit in the sauna to heat their bodies and then jump into an ice-cold pool.

My recommendation is that anyone taking a hot shower should finish up with a cold shower. In this way, the body will become much more adept at dealing with the stresses of environmental temperature fluctuations. For years, I started my day with a cold shower, and I did not have one day of sickness, a cold or flu. I mention this way of dealing with allergies in order to show that, even in extreme cases, water can be effective very quickly.

Question: Can I quit asthma and allergy medications if I increase my water and salt intake?

Answer: On no account should you abruptly cut off the use of your medications. You should begin taking more water at the same time as you continue your medication, until your need for medication decreases. You will then be able to reduce the use of the normally prescribed inhalant or antihistamine medications until you no longer need them. Keep the doctor in charge of your treatment informed.

In obstinate and truly drug-dependent cases of asthma and allergies, increased water intake will improve the patient's response to the medications being prescribed until he or she becomes free of their need. Curing a long-standing condition produced by dehydration might take longer than anticipated. The extra time is needed to reassemble some of the functions that get lost due to the "chemical cascades" that delete some manufacturing systems that have become "idle" because of water shortage and irregular delivery of primary materials.

Question: Will plain tap water do?

Answer: The choice of water should not become a limiting factor to drinking it. So long as tap water contains no lead, mercury, pesticides, or other dangerous chemicals or bacteria, it should become your fluid of choice. You should not worry about its "hardness." The calcium that is dissolved in the water will even serve a useful purpose. It will help meet your body's need for calcium. If the smell of chlorine is too much, fill an open-top jug, leave it exposed to air, and the chlorine, which is a gas, will evaporate in less than a half hour. The water will be sweet and ready to drink.

It is becoming a vogue to advocate drinking distilled water. The claim that distilled water is better for you than other types of water may prove to be based on the commercial aims of its manufacturers. In any case, the body filters the water we drink through its cell membranes and uses "almost distilled" water inside its cells. You do not need to worry about this issue; the human body has been designed to take nothing for granted. Moreover, a constant use of distilled water may, in the long run, take some minerals from the teeth as these are its first point of contact with something it can dissolve. In any event, water is dis-tilled only as long as it is in the bottle. As soon as it enters the body, it mixes with whatever is in the intestinal tract—remnants of food, and bacterial and intestinal flora's byproducts. One can use distilled water if no other natural source for water is avail-able, such as when on board a ship at sea. Operating a distiller for drinking water is an expensive and cumbersome process.

Question: Should I watch for any complications?

Answer: With increased water intake that causes increased urine production, there may be an associated loss of salt, miner-als and water-soluble vitamins. Supplementing your daily salt and vitamin intake will be necessary. If you develop cramps, you should assume that the salt in your diet is not sufficient for your body's needs. You should add some salt to your diet as long as you stick to taking more water. Salt acts as a natural antihista-mine. It also helps break up sticky mucus and make it more fluid so that it separates more easily from the lung tissue and can be coughed up. Salt shortage in the diet can be a contributing factor in asthma attacks. Developing a feeling of nausea when you drink water is a sign of salt shortage in your body.

Q **uestion:** Where can I get more information about the curative properties of water?

Answer: You can learn more about the intricate functions of water in my book, *Your Body's Many Cries for Water.* This book has been designed to provide the general public with some crucial insights into the newly discovered emergency and crisis thirst signals of the human body. If you wish to know more about chronic dehydration and its potential for disease production in your body, this book shares with you all that is now known about this newly discovered topic.

The information in the book reveals why water by itself is the only nature-ordained medicine for some of our everyday "disease" conditions. The scientific background to this book is my extensive research into the relationship of stress and water metabolism of the body, including the water regulatory roles of the neurotransmitter histamine. I have had the honor and the pleasure of having introduced this topic at different international conferences, in scientific publications, in media interviews, in self-treatment books, and at public lectures.

You can also listen to my ten-hour, audiotape seminar, *Water: Rx for a Healthier Pain-Free Life,* or watch my two-hour lecture video, *Cure Pain and Prevent Cancer.*

"In the arts of life man invents
nothing; but in the arts of death
he outdoes Nature herself, and
produces by chemistry and
machinery all the slaughter of
plague, pestilence and famine."

George Bernard Shaw

5

How Water Cured Their Asthma and Allergies

The following stories should make you think along the line of my researched findings. In the testimonials that follow, you will read from people whose asthma and allergies were cured by increased water and salt intake.

Jeremy Christopher was eight years old when I first heard about his asthma problem in 1995. He is the son of Dr. Cheryl Brown-Christopher, a medical doctor. Jeremy had suffered from severe allergies and asthma for three to four years. By the end of March 1995, he had developed extreme discomfort from a severely congested upper respiratory tract. He was constantly coughing as a complication of his asthma, and he had severe shortness of breath. He was on two different medications (Benadryl and Albuterol inhaler—Figure 9), which caused drowsiness. They made him uncommunicative and withdrawn from group activity in class. As a result, his school grades were poor.

Dr. Brown-Christopher obtained the book, *Your Body's Many Cries for Water,* and, after reading its chapter on allergies and asthma, she contacted me to discuss her son's problem. We came to the conclusion that Jeremy should stop the intake of all manufactured beverages and substitute them with about six to eight cups of plain water a day. He should drink two cups of water before each meal and before exercise. He should also consume one half teaspoon of salt a day to offset its loss in the increased urine produced by the added 10 full cups of water. *This is a rough ratio of water and salt intake per day—a half teaspoon of salt for every 10 cups of water.* Salt intake is critical for asthma prevention.

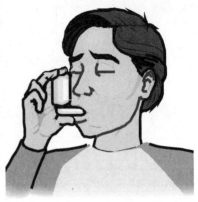

Figure 9

The result in Dr. Brown-Christopher's own words: "Within three to four days he showed dramatic improvement; he no longer had severe and excessive mucus production, his coughing had virtually stopped, and his sneezing and other allergy symptoms were totally gone.... Therefore we discontinued his Benadryl and Albuterol and continued his hydration.... Not only have his symptoms cleared subjectively, but in terms of objective findings, his peak flow volumes have been within normal range (this means the lungs are aerated normally).... His constant medication-induced drowsiness has disappeared and as a result he is more alert, and his school grades have improved." Jeremy's lung capacity increased from 60 percent of the normal average, even with the intake of medications, to 120 percent of the normal with no medications. Dr. Christopher's letters are printed on the next pages.

Of the 17 million children like Jeremy who suffer from asthma, a few thousand of them die every year. These children can be cured just as easily as Jeremy. All they and their families need to understand is that, in reality, asthmatics are so thirsty that for them breathing has become difficult—one of the human body's crisis calls for water.

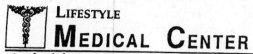

LIFESTYLE
MEDICAL CENTER

Family Medicine • Reconstruction Therapy for Back, Knee, Hand and Joint Pain • Varicose Vein Therapy

Dr. Batmanghelidj   May 24, 1995
2146 Kings Garden Way
Falls Church, VA 22043

Reference: Jeremy Christopher

Dear Dr. Batmanghelidj:

I am writing to thank you for your kind assistance in treating Jeremy's allergies. As you know, Jeremy is my eight year-old son who suffered for the last 3-4 years with severe allergy symptoms related to allergic rhinitis and asthma.

More Recently he has had significant coryza and coughing which is associated with his asthma. On about the 28th of April 1995, we began a program of rehydration involving his drinking two cups of water before food or exercise and excluding all other fluids. In addition, he consumes a half teaspoon of salt which is added to his food to offset the increased water intake.

Within 3-4 days he showed dramatic improvement; he no longer had severe and excessive mucus production, his coughing had virtually stopped, and his sneezing and other allergy symptoms were totally gone. Therefore we discontinued his Benadryl and Albuterol and continued his hydration program.

Jeremy has been following this program now for approximately four and a half weeks, spending almost four weeks off his medication and is doing quite well. Not only have his symptoms cleared subjectively, but in terms of objective findings, his peak flow volumes have been within normal range. His constant medication-induced drowsiness has disappeared and as a result he is more alert, and his school grades have improved.

Therefore I want to emphasize how effective this treatment has been for Jeremy and I wish you well in sharing this cost effective and very efficacious program with others.

Once again Dr. Batmanghelidj, I thank you for advising me on the new treatment program of Jeremy's allergies and asthma.

Very truly yours,

Cheryl Brown-Christopher, M.D.

1419 Forest Drive • Suite #202 • Annapolis • Maryland 21403 • (410) 268-5005

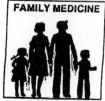
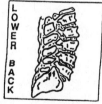
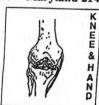
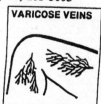

Dr. Cheryl Brown-Christopher recently sent me an update on Jeremy's condition.

August 3, 1999
Re: Jeremy Christopher

Dear Dr. Batmanghelidj,

Once again, I am writing to thank you and update you on the results from your precious advice regarding water intake and allergies for my son, Jeremy. As you may recall, four years ago, Jeremy at the age of eight had severe symptoms of allergic rhinitis, including runny eyes, continuous sneezing, coughing, and reduced mental concentration; he additionally had been diagnosed with asthma. Inhalers and antihistamines provided minimal benefit, and plans were in progress to begin desensitization injections (allergy shots). Fortunately, during this period of time, we met you and you advised me to begin Jeremy on your protocol of drinking 6-8 glasses of water daily along with a fi teaspoon of salt per day. Within two weeks, Jeremy's symptoms had completely resolved and his peak flowmeter readings increased over 50%. In essence, Jeremy's lung volume readings became normal and his hayfever cleared without medication!

Jeremy is now a twelve-year-old, upcoming seventh grader, who has never taken allergy shots and is doing well after four years of following the "Batman water protocol." To be candid, Dr. Batmanghelidj, my son will periodically drink soda or juices and experience very short-lived flare-up of sneezing when exposed to ragweed, pollen, or dust concurrently with drinking these beverages. Fortunately, the symptoms clear very rapidly with his ingesting two glasses of water and fi teaspoon of salt or salty foods.

My husband and I continue to monitor Jeremy's peak flowmeter readings only sporadically now, as he has been asymptomatic with respect to asthma for four years and his readings are always normal. I have been so impressed with these results, Dr. Batmanghelidj, that I advise every patient in my orthopedic and family practice to follow your protocol. I have seen remarkable improvements in patients with allergies— including asthma—attention deficit disorder, diabetes, back pain, arthritis, hypertension, and many other chronic illnesses who follow your protocol.

Dr. Batman, in my opinion, Jeremy is cured of asthma and allergic rhinitis as a result of your outstanding research on the benefits of water. This breakthrough approach to allergies and other chronic diseases is effective, convenient, and affordable to all. I am deeply grateful to you as both a mother and a physician. May God bless you in your continued efforts to spread the word to all.

> *Sincerely,*
> *Cheryl Brown-Christopher, M.D.*
> *Diplomate, AAPM, FAAFP*

☞ ☞ ☞ ☞ ☞

Jose Rivera, M.D., developed adult-onset allergies and asthma when he was in college. At times he would get such severe attacks that he would need hospitalization for his suffocation and shocked state. He was allergic to cats more severely than other things. Apparently, he would never step into a house where a cat was kept as a pet. Before accepting an invitation, he would ask if they kept a cat. Such was the state of his body sensitivity to some allergens.

One day in 1994, while he was talking to me on the telephone, I noticed his repeated dry and gasping coughs. This was when I learned about his asthma. I asked him to drink a glass of water and put a pinch of salt on his tongue while we were talking on the telephone. His words: "As you recall, I was having a coughing spell that interrupted my work and, as you directed, the putting of some granules of salt on my tongue not only calmed my coughing but took it away. My nurses commented on my not coughing some five minutes later." In Dr. Rivera, his cough was the telltale indicator of his asthma that had given him more problems than he could ever think of as a modern, well-trained physician.

For the past four years, he has been free of asthma and allergies. He seems not to fear cats any more. He can now visit friends who have cats in their homes. He now treats his asthmatic patients with water and some added salt intake. For him, the initial cough when he comes across a cat means he is not drinking enough water. The cough clears up as soon as he takes water and some salt. He is a good example that when we start on our needed daily water intake, we manifest our critical need for water by our own body's individual "signature tune"—in Dr. Rivera's case, the initial telltale cough of an impending asthma attack. Here are his own words, on pages 61 and 62.

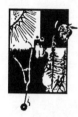

VON KIEL FAMILY MEDICINE & WELLNESS CENTER

Erik Von Kiel, D.O.   *Board Certified Family Practice with emphasis on Preventive Medicine*

Liberty Square Medical Cent.
501 North 17th Street • Suite :
Allentown, PA 18104
(610) 776-7639

Jose A. Rivera M.D.   1/6/95
Lecturer/Member Advisory Board
International Federation of Holistic Medicine

Dr. F. Batmanghelidj
Global Health Solutions
Falls Church, VA. 22043

Dear Dr. Batmanghelidj

This letter is in appreciatiion for the information that you have presented concerning water dehydration and asthma. As you recall I have had adult onset asthma since I was in college and have had many bouts of anaphylaxis which were life threatening.

Due to the information that you have provided I have been able to ameliorate and cure my own asthma with water and salt intake. I have been asthma free for approximately 1.5 years and have not had any reactions to the allergens of the past.

The information has been most helpful in making me aware of when and how to drink water and take salt inorder to hydrate myself and prevent any recurrence of asthma.

Also, I have been able to advise other patients with respiratory and allergen problems in how to increase their water and salt intake safely, and to my amazement the amelioration has been dramatic.

Thank you sir for giving me and others the breath of life thru something so simple as water and salt.

Sincerely,

Jose A. Rivera M.D.

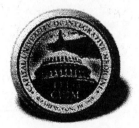

Jose A. Rivera MD.
Associate Professor
Capital University of Integrative Medicine
1131 8th St. NE.
Washington, DC. 20002
Auricular Acupuncture Medicine
2323 St. Matthew's Rd.
Orangeburg, SC. 29118
803-531-6005
Esoj@Earthlink.net

Dr. F. Batmanghelidj   2-14-2000
Global Health Solutions
Falls Church, Virginia

Dear Dr. Batmanghelidj
Since my letter of 1-6-95, I have been asthma free for approximately 4 years since
initially being introduced to your prescription for health in taking water and salt as
preventive measures that also cured my asthma attacks. Remembering to watch for
signs of stress and fatigue, which can induce bronchial constriction for water
preservation and rationing. This is very important since it is during these times that
one is unaware of what is really happening physiologically.
Listening to one's own body can enable one to prevent what was once a common
occurrence; bronchial constriction which later leads to asthma.
It is through these simple directions of hydrating the body with water and regulating
the salt levels that one can begin to prevent and cure asthma and heal a body in need
of better hydration.
Your prescription for health is certainly a constant reminder to a recovering asthmatic.
Thank you for your attention and constant help.
Sincerely,

Jose A. Rivera MD.

Michael Peck is in his 50s. He suffered from allergies and eventually asthma since childhood. Later in life he became overweight and developed high blood pressure. His allergies were so bad that he needed to check the daily pollen count before deciding if he could step out of the house. Thirteen years ago he became aware of the curative properties of water in asthma and allergy. He started regulating his daily water intake and stopped drinking tea and coffee. When everyone in the office took coffee, he drank hot water. Since then, Michael has not had any asthma attacks. His allergy became much less troublesome, almost to the point of being nonexistent. He no longer bothers with the pollen count. He has been free of allergy and asthma attacks since he started to regulate his daily water intake. He considers himself cured of these health problems. In my opinion, he is cured as long as he sticks to his water intake routine.

MICRO INVESTMENTS, INC.

....

25 March 1992

Dr. F. Batmanghelidj
Foundation For The Simple In Medicine
2146 Kings Garden Way
Falls Church, Va. 22043

Dear Fereydoon,

This letter is a testimony to the merits of water as an essential part of the daily dietary requirements for good health. I have been following your recommendations for nearly five years, and have found myself taking for granted the positive effects of water intake.

When I first started on the program I was overweight, with high blood pressure and suffering from asthma and allergies, which I have had since a small child. I had been receiving treatment for these conditions. Today, I have my weight and blood pressure under control (weight loss of approximately 30 pounds and a 10 point drop in blood pressure). The program reduced the frequency of asthma and allergy related problems, to the point of practical nonexistence. Additionally, there were other benefits, I experienced fewer colds and flus, and generally with less severity.

I introduced this program to my wife, who had been on blood pressure medication for the past four years, and through increased water intake has recently been able to eliminate her medication.

Thanks again for your program,

Michael Peck

Nearly seven years later, Mr. Peck reported that he continued to enjoy the benefits of good health.

Dr. Fereydoon Batmanghelidj
2146 Kings Garden Way
Falls Church, VA 22043
January 21, 1999

Dear Fereydoon:

I would like to give you a quick update on the success of the hydration program I have been following for the last several years. I am almost totally free from the severe allergic reactions I suffered from all my life. When I do have a reaction it is mild and short, and I enjoy the side benefit that I am almost never sick with the flu and/or colds. The most beneficial effect of this program has been to keep my hypertension condition within acceptable parameters. Your advice several years ago has significantly improved the quality and duration of my life. I am a grateful and devoted student of your principles of hydration.

I would like to thank you for your continued devotion to the study of the healing properties of proper body hydration.

Sincerely,
Michael A. Peck

☞ ☞ ☞ ☞ ☞

Nathaniel C. is a young man in his 20s. He suffered from asthma since childhood. On several occasions he developed attacks that needed immediate professional attention at the emergency department of the nearest hospital. In recent years, one of these attacks was so severe that he needed to be hospitalized. Consequently, in constant fear of a repeat of these attacks, Nathaniel kept his inhaler with him always and used it frequently, possibly more often than prescribed. A good morning to him would mean just a few puffs from his inhaler. He could not endure smoky rooms. He could not go through a business meeting without the support of his inhaler, nor could he exercise with the same abandon and pleasure as his friends. For Nathaniel, fear and the constant threat of another attack preoccupied his mind and punctuated the day's activity.

When he became aware of the topic of my research—chronic dehydration—he wanted to know if his asthma could also be cured with water. He was surprised when I informed him that asthma was caused mainly by chronic dehydration. After he adjusted his daily water intake and reduced his coffee intake, his breathing became more comfortable. He could go longer hours without needing his "puffs of medication." He was able to reduce and eventually do away with his inhaler. He has been virtually free of his asthma and its associated fears for the past seven years.

Annette C. Penny is a journalist and public relations consultant whose husband had suffered from asthma for a number of years. Mr. "P." was on various medications for his asthma that had so incapacitated him that he had become almost confined to his house and his room, with medications on hand at all times. Life had become unbearable for both of them: for her, the unbearable anxiety of his impending death, and for him, the drudgery of life in constant suffocation. Such was the quality of their lives before the morning she met me at a Rotary Club meeting. She asked my opinion about her husband's asthma. I told her not to wait until she got home, but to telephone her husband and tell him to begin drinking plenty of water immediately.

It did not take more than a few days of following the instructions I gave his wife for him to see the miraculous improvement in his breathing and in his capacity to move and talk. He did not need to use the nebulizer he had rented. Mrs. Penny was very impressed with the unexpected results of her husband's response to simple water. She kept referring to it as "a miracle." She even wrote an article about it that was published in the *Journal Messenger* of Manassas, VA, in September 1993. (This date is given to show how long the information on the cure of asthma has been in the public domain, and yet we still have to fight to spread it.)

Such was the positive impact of regulating daily water intake in one of many millions of desperate asthmatics. Not only did increased daily water intake cause improvement in this particular man's quality and expectancy of life, indirectly it also relieved his devastated wife.

Priscilla Preston's letter to me begins: "Imagine having to sleep in an upright position for almost a year, struggling for each breath and suffering from countless asthma and panic attacks nightly! That was me until five months ago! On March 27, 1993, I was hospitalized with a severe asthma attack and developed bronchial pneumonia! My blood gases registered 40 and I was in a life-threatening situation!" She had heard about my book, *Your Body's Many Cries for Water*, which she bought and read. All she needed to know was the cause of asthma—dehydration. Armed with the new information on asthma, she was cured of the disease. In her own words: "As of this date, October 31, 1994, I am no longer on any medication for asthma! I have not used an inhaler or medication of any sort for more than five months! When I start any sort of mild wheezing, I just drink a glass of water and take a little salt and I am fine." She also lost 45 pounds of excess weight.

Please bear in mind that asthma is not a "disease;" it is a drastic complication of water shortage in the body. It is the out-come of a very strict drought management program in the body. Any time an asthmatic does not drink enough water or take enough salt, his or her predisposition to asthma attacks will come back. You cannot be lazy about regularly drinking adequate water and taking some salt to replenish that lost salt in the urine or in perspiration and then expect asthma to stay away. Recurrence of symptoms became the painful experience of Mr. "P.", mentioned earlier. He decreased his water intake and after a few weeks his asthma recurred. He would also take the odd alco-holic drink that dehydrated his body even more.

Let me tell you a story and then I will tell you more about Priscilla Preston.

"Mullah" is a folklore character in Persian literature. He is sincere, sometimes intelligent, but often a simpleton. He is easily tricked and falls for the simplest of scams, even his own! One day he went to buy bread at his favorite bakery and found himself at the end of a long line. He suddenly had an idea to clear the line and not to have to wait to buy bread. Addressing the people ahead of him in the line, he said, "The bakery down the road is giving people free bread." This utterance from a respectable-looking man in his teacher/holy man gown had the desired effect. All those in line rushed down the road towards the other bakery. You would have thought Mullah would have seized the opportunity to now buy his bread. No! Instead, he got caught up in the excitement of the people running to the other bakery and he forgot that it was his scam that had caused the rush. He said to himself, "There must be something to it if all those people are going there." Without hesitation, he rushed after the others. By the time he reached the other bakery he was again at the end of the line.

What does this story have to do with Priscilla? She is certainly intelligent, but like Mullah, she fell for a scam—in her case, the false information put out by the pharmaceutical industry.

In search of a more responsible job, she landed a position with a pharmaceutical company in Texas. She became the company's director of sales for some regions of Texas, and eventually became vice president of sales for North Carolina. Unfortunately she bought into the teaching of the sick care system that salt is bad for hypertension and she began to abstain from salt, one of the most vital elements to the human body. As time went on, she began to experience shortness of breath and coughing until her full-blown asthma recurred. She had been free of asthma for nearly five years. Now she again suffers from it and is on medication.

When there is shortage of salt in the diet and there is increased water intake, the body becomes truly salt deficient. Increased urine production washes away the mineral reserves of the body, with salt at the top of the list. Salt, especially unrefined salt from the ocean, contains many vital elements that balance the mineral content of the blood, including the element sodium.

A salt-deficient body is actually in a state of severe drought. However, when only water is taken in large amounts, the cells, particularly the brain cells, become overhydrated and subject to irreversible damage, possibly resulting in death. Salt expands the water volume held in blood and serum. From this "ocean of water" held outside the cells, water is filtered and injected into the vital cells, offsetting the effect of drought inside the cells. It is my view that asthmatics fall short of the safe level of the ocean of water outside the cells and trigger the drought management program we call asthma.

Asthmatics should understand that the design of their bodies is such that, in water shortage and persistent dehydration, their air passages close down to prevent water from evaporating into the air that is breathed out. This is a mechanism of drought management that is installed in their bodies. It might reveal itself before any other sign of dehydration.

Dr. Ruurd van Roorda, an asthma expert at De Weezenlanden Hospital in Zwolle, Holland, followed a few hundred children with asthma for more than 15 years and showed that over 70 percent of these children continued to have breathing problems even when they were well into their second decade of life.

It has become apparent that, even if asthmatics become symptom-free for a short while, they tend to be revisited by the problem in their later years. In other words, asthmatics are seldom completely free of their breathing problems. This is illustrated by a report published in *The New York Times* on January 4, 1994, on a research project in Holland. This is the reason why asthma is a very serious health problem when only treated with chemical medications. These medications do not correct the basic dehydration of the body that has triggered the phase of drought management designed to prolong life a short while longer until more water enters the body.

Any time an asthmatic experiences difficulty in breathing— the dry cough signals imminent danger—and thinks an asthma attack is in the making, he or she should quickly take two or three glasses of water, one after another, and then put a pinch of salt on the tongue. Salt acts as an effective, natural antihistamine that, through the salt-sensing nerves located on the tongue, will act directly on the brain and help make breathing easier and more effective.

Histamine is an important neurotransmitter that manages water distribution and its intake in the body. It also rations water during drought management, hence its shutting down of the bronchioles in asthma. People with asthma need to drink no less than 10 eight-ounce glasses of water throughout every day of their lives. They should also take about a half teaspoon of salt for every 10 glasses of water, every day. This is about a quarter teaspoon of salt for every quart of water. Salt should be added to their food. A salt-free or very-low-salt diet is absolutely stupid. In my opinion, a low-salt diet is a major contributing factor to the onset of asthma. That is to say, asthma is caused by both a water and salt shortage in the body!

An asthmatic who is under medication should not stop its use, but should take water and salt together until he or she feels confident to go without medication. The body understands when the level of its water and salt content is adequate to get out of drought management mode and relieves the anxiety that is associated with asthma. Complete discontinuance of medication should be approved by the physician in charge. If the physician does not understand the relationship of asthma to dehydration, *it is your moral responsibility* to share your newly gained insight with the doctor. If he or she chooses to ignore the information, change your doctor. A physician who does not understand the locked-in relationship of water and histamine, and refuses to learn about it, can cause more damage than do good, not only to you but to other unsuspecting and trusting persons.

In the following pages, I have chosen to present a typical case history of ongoing chronic dehydration in childhood and to show how, in the "fourth dimension of time," various other conditions produced by dehydration reveal themselves, step-by-step and stage-by-stage. Because we don't realize that each and every one of the health problems I mentioned at the beginning of the book are part and parcel of the same water shortage that is not recognized and corrected, we coin different labels to define one or other aspect of the main problem, which is drought inside the cells.

Medicine of today resembles the outcome of 10 blind people's attempt to describe an elephant by each feeling a different part of its anatomy. They do not realize that all the parts belong to the same great animal. The blind-to-dehydration doctors have similarly composed reams of verbiage about what "they have seen" without realizing why they saw it. They certainly do not appreciate that they have described the same thing—dehydration—but have given it a variety of different disease labels.

Andrew Bauman's story will one day be considered a classic case of a young man who suffered from dehydration from childhood and lived to demonstrate the relationship between persistent water shortage and many different serious health problems. He also demonstrates how water can actually cure reversible conditions and ease the problems of irreversible ones.

His life story also reflects my deep-felt concern about asthma and allergies in children. With the right kind of treatment, children can be saved naturally and at no cost; yet, with the currently practiced protocols, children are doomed to a lifetime of suffering and an unnatural, early death.

Read Andrew Bauman's letter and judge for yourself. His letter is long; however, it shows what can go wrong in a person who does not understand the true indicators of dehydration in the human body.

November 13, 1998

Dear Dr. Batmanghelidj:

My name is Andrew J. Bauman, IV, and I am 42 years young, yet at age 34 I felt and looked like I was at least 44! Most of my life has been spent battling illness and disease, whereas now I celebrate each moment of each day with a renewed vigor and vitality. I used to be chronically dehydrated and now I know better.

I was born on October 29, 1956 in Taylor, PA, in a small hospital near Scranton in Northeast Pennsylvania. My parents lovingly cared for me—including having me vaccinated. I was reared on infant formula and, later, on cereal, juices, and a small amount of water when I would cry from colic. After my first polio vaccine, I became mysteriously paralyzed from the waist down. Specialists were puzzled yet diagnosed "Aborted Polio." It left as suddenly as it appeared. When I received a booster dose of the vaccine at around age five in first grade, the paralysis returned. Months of hospitalization and bed rest resulted in my gaining weight. I mostly ate my meals and had visitors, drank soda and some water now and then—and once again the paralyzation disappeared.

When I began third grade—around eight years old—my allergic afflictions and symptoms had begun. I had problems with frequent dry coughs. I began experiencing some difficulties with breathing, itchy and watery eyes, and fatigue when I was around freshly cut lawns from springtime until autumn. When I was a junior in high school, I experienced blackouts from allergies. Sometime around 1979, I saw a specialist who did tests and diagnosed me with allergies and asthma. I was approximately 23 years old. I was treated with allergy shots and inhalers.

The treatments just seemed to make things worse. My lips

were always dry and cracked. At that time of my life I was drinking about two to four cups of coffee per day along with a few glasses of soda and some tea and alcohol. I would have an occasional glass of water during the day. The allergies and asthma stayed with me until 1996 when my water intake was up to about two to three quarts a day. I no longer struggle with allergies or asthma.

My problems with diabetes began at age 14. I was diagnosed as an insulin-dependent or "juvenile" diabetic. It was then that I began drinking diet beverages including those with caffeine. My water intake at that time was still only around two to four glasses a day and I was drinking tea and started drinking coffee. The diabetes resulted in many hospitalizations over the years. By the mid-1980s I had problems with diabetic neuropathy which was causing my legs to swell. I was scheduled to have dye injected into my legs to perform a diagnostic scan after a Doppler radar study showed some apparent blockages in the veins in my legs. The dye injections caused my veins to burst which made the swelling get worse. I was then diagnosed with "venous insufficiency." In 1994, I was told that my legs would probably have to be removed within a year or so.

While attempting to get on a diabetic insulin supply trial, the initial examination revealed that the retinas in my eyes had blood vessels that were bleeding (diabetic retinopathy). I began receiving a series of laser surgeries over the next 15 years to attempt to seal the leaky vessels and to attempt to prevent any new vessel growth. This reduced my peripheral and night vision. In 1992, I developed an enlarged yet benign prostate gland and my kidneys began showing signs of deterioration. In 1993, I began experiencing some potency difficulties. In 1994, I began seeing a natural or homeopathic physician who, besides treating me with alternative medicine, advised me to increase my water intake. My intake of insulin was around 95 units daily.

In 1976, many immune system problems began developing. I graduated from high school in 1974 and went away to college. In

1976, I got a job as a mental health worker while going to school. I met my wife and, while dating, working full time, and going to school part time, I developed "Infectious Mononucleosis."

My wife and I were married in 1977 and I continued to struggle with many infections and illnesses as well as losing my job in 1978. In 1979, during one of my then frequent hospital stays, I was diagnosed with "mono" again! The doctors insisted that I shouldn't have "mono" again and began consulting with specialists. I received an influenza vaccine and was discharged—only to be readmitted a day later with a fever of 106 deg F. I was undergoing many tests, however nothing much was showing up at that time.

After many tests for severe abdominal pain, I was told that I "grew a second spleen that was attached to my spleen and that the second one was also functioning." That year I was visiting someone and drank unpasteurized milk and ended up in the hospital again with a bacterial infection of the intestinal tract. "Brucellosis and Proteus—ox-19" was the diagnosis and I was on yet more antibiotics.

During 1980 or 1981, I developed another case of "mono" and was admitted to the hospital again, diabetic control problems were a constant battle for me. An Infectious Disease specialist discovered that a number of special antibodies against foreign agents were also affected, which the doctors suggested were related to the problems with my allergies and asthma, as well as my frequent infections.

The 1980s were filled with many hospitalizations, illnesses, job losses, and stress-related problems. It was then that I was diagnosed with allergies to penicillin and tetracycline, began developing hypertension, was diagnosed with chronic fatigue syndrome, lymphoid hyperplasia (over-stressed immune system), arthritis, bursitis, fibromyalgia, and gastroporesis or acid reflux problems, and bowel problems.

I also developed a benign tumor on the left flank of my back.

I developed a nodule on my thyroid area and was diagnosed with lead, cadmium, and aluminum poisoning which was also found in a landfill I lived near. I was overweight and developed sleep apnea. Tests showed that I stopped breathing over 300 times in a six-hour period and had "narcolepsy." I could fall asleep in a short period of time. I had surgery to attempt to correct the sleep apnea, and I wore a tracheotomy tube in my neck to help me breathe at night, and slept with a breathing machine to keep my airway open. During the 80s I still only drank a few glasses of water, yet consumed large amounts of coffee, saccharin, and eventually NutraSweet. In 1987, I was declared "disabled."

In 1992, at 36 years old, I looked and felt like I was in my late forties and felt worse than I looked. I began using natural supplements with vitamins, herbs, and other natural medical techniques. The homeopathic doctor's advice was to increase my water consumption and decrease my caffeine intake as well. I had lost the feeling in my feet, was always tired and achy, depressed, and had little hope.

I began to drink more water and reduced my caffeine intake somewhat, and by 1995 I began to feel and look much better. Yet I was still only consuming a quart to a quart and a half daily, and not flushing all the caffeine out of my system, nor was I using sea salt.

In September of 1995, that lump on my left flank turned red, began itching, and enlarging. My family physician removed it and sent it away for study. In October, I was diagnosed with cutaneous B cell lymphoma. Twenty-six new tumors had grown on my back where there was one, and I was sent to a major hospital where I was told that lymphatic cancer on the skin surface was rare and that not much research was done yet on it.

I went for a gallium scan and it revealed that my entire body surface glowed positive for cancer cells. The flank of my back was brighter white or "hyper-positive," as was the middle of my chest where two melanomas were previously removed. I was advised to receive localized radiation and "as tumors appeared we would radiate them too or I could travel to Philadelphia and have my entire body surface radiated." They began to radiate my back which began giving me third-degree burns. I refused total body radiation and, midway through my radiation, my homeo-pathic physician began using a natural cleansing therapy. The cancer specialist had advised me to try anything and to "pull out all the stops," as well as to "get my affairs in order." I increased my water consumption and took supplements and natural treatments.

In November of 1995, while traveling in search of an answer, I had to buy tires for my car. At the auto parts store where I was looking for tires, I was introduced to Bob Butts who exposed me to your water cure program and advised me to stick to it very seriously to get cured. I now began to seriously increase my water intake but was still leery of increasing salt intake due to the traditional medical contra-indications for its perceived high blood pressure problems. Later I learned of the error of that thinking and began to increase my salt intake too.

In March of 1996, I went for another gallium scan which revealed that there was not a single sign of cancer glowing pos-itive on my entire body. Doctors thought there was an error in the gallium scan, but my homeopath and I knew that I was healing. Drinking more water, reducing caffeine, a change in dietary habits, natural medicine, and faith had brought me home. I acknowledge God's presence in me and remember the scripture, "I am the living waters." He called me and you "the salt of the earth," and tells us that we are "one in spirit."

Since then, I've been constantly improving in my health. I no longer have two spleens, but one that is normal in size and func-tion. Now I lick sea salt off my palm in the morning before my first glass of water and use salt liberally. I drink about 1.5 gal-lons of water a day and take some supplements as well as eating a lot of whole grains and fresh fruits and vegetables. My waist used to be a size 43 and now is a size 36. I weighed 249 pounds, now I weigh 210 and have solid muscle mass. My complexion and appearance are those of a man in his early thirties and my potency of a man in his twenties.

My ankles are no longer swollen and new pulses, yes, new pulses, have developed where once they were dead. I no longer take any medications for all those problems, whereas I used to be on at least 15 prescriptions at a time. My insulin needs are down from 95 units a day to 35-45 units a day. I no longer suffer with "chronic infections" or fatigue—I sleep 6-8 hours a day instead of 12-14. It is rare for me to take an antibiotic, whereas I seemed to be constantly taking them before. I don't have allergies or asthma or gastroporesis (acid reflux) any more. I no longer suffer from arthritis, bursitis, or bowel problems. At the time of my last stress test, my Doctor who is younger than I am told me that I was in better shape than he was. The high blood pressure is constantly improving. No more thyroid nodule, I sleep better, and no more heavy metal toxicity. I have a new lease on life.

My prayers have been answered. God led me to a natural way to heal my body, my mind, and my spirit. I am living a new life now with a balance of water, salt, minerals, supplements, good nutrition, and continued improvements in my quality of life. I am truly blessed.

You have my permission to use this letter in any way you think will help spread the news of the medicinal value of water in medical treatment procedures.

> *Sincerely,*
> *Andrew J. Bauman, IV*
> *Pennsylvania*

☞ ☞ ☞ ☞ ☞

Who would have thought there were so many miracles of health and wellness in simple water? Who could have thought that lack of water flow in the body could cause so many health problems that were reversible? Mr. Bauman's account is one of the first where water has been shown to have medicinal value in the treatment of cancer. I will discuss his letter extensively in my next book, *ABC of Cancer and Depression*.

Let us see what we learn from the letter from a Dutch doctor.

Hans C. Moolenburgh, M.D.
2012 LN Haarlem
Oranjeplein 11
Netherlands
3 February 1997

Dear Doctor Batmanghelidj,

Once in a blue moon one comes across a really revolutionary book. It happens so seldom that those moments stand out as highlights. Your book, "Your Body's Many Cries for Water," is such a book and moreover I finally know who to thank for my recovery. This of course sounds strange, so I will tell you.

In the summer of 1993 I was on vacation with my wife in Spain. On a hot day we went to the beach and paddled around in our rubber boat. Afterwards, at the hottest moment of the day, we climbed the steep rocky path to our car and there and then my breath left me. I was 68 at that time so I was not too astonished, but the strange thing was that my breath did not return.

Ten days later we came back from that holiday and my breath was still somewhere on that rocky path. At least, it did not come home with me. I resumed my practice and still I was out of breath. I had X-rays taken as I had treated a woman with an open T.B., but nothing. When, in the fall, my breath had still not come back, a doctor in New York gave me a telephone call and he asked me: "You talk differently. What is the matter with your breath?" I told him about it and he said: "You did not drink enough. You're the victim of a bronchial constriction and this is caused by your body trying to save your water supplies." I had never heard that one before, but I took his advice and began to drink 8 glasses of water a day, and in one week all my breathlessness had evaporated as if it had never been there.

Since then, I realized that in my youth I drank a lot of water but somewhere along the road I had lost the habit, so I began to drink more pure water (as my friend had stressed). Everything went well until this winter. It was so extremely cold in December that I just stopped drinking all that cold water for a while. This happened to coincide with a rather strenuous dental repair which was rather painful and suddenly I developed gastritis with a tongue as white as snow. I suddenly remembered that my New York friend had told me that another pathway the body chooses to stop losing water is to close the pylorus. I straight away started taking 8 glasses of water again (luckily the cold weather had lessened considerably) and within four days my stomach was healed, much to the surprise of a young colleague who had never heard of gastritis healing so fast.

You asked for corroborating evidence in your book so this is why I send you this lengthy letter.

I have been a medical practitioner for 27 years and after that (since 1981) I left general practice and now I am a consultant on allergy, food and chemical intolerances and holistic treatment for cancer. I have already used the water treatment for asthma in my extensive children's practice (half of my patients are under 10 years old) and I definitely see results. I can say from personal experience, both on myself and in my practice, that I can affirm what you have found.

> *Yours sincerely,*
> *Hans C. Moolenburgh, M.D.*

☞ ☞ ☞ ☞ ☞

My message on asthma is getting around. It has even traveled from one continent to another, and the person who testifies to its efficacy is another seasoned medical doctor. I think the New

York doctor had come across my book or Sam Biser's interview with me on asthma in 1993. Martha Avelar, whose letter appears below, had read the same newsletter interview by Sam Biser.

Martha Avelar
3521 Vanderbilt Court
Garland, Texas 75043
September 13, 1993

Dear Dr. Batmanghelidj,

Again, I wish to thank you for helping me to better appreciate the importance of water to my health.

In May of this year, I acquired a sinus infection followed by bronchitis in June. Both were treated medically and apparently successfully. The following month, while vacationing in the high country (8,000 to 10,000 feet elevation) of New Mexico, I developed difficulty in breathing to the point that I cut my vacation short to consult with my doctor.

The problem seemed to be shortness of breath or insufficient intake of air. My doctor immediately referred me to the hospital for a series of tests in view of my breathing problem and the previous sinus and bronchitis that I had experienced. In the hospital my lungs were X rayed, oxygen content in my blood tested, EKGed, stress tested, heart monitored for 24 hours, and my lungs were scanned. Tests revealed nothing. On the third day I was released and was prescribed Xanax to be taken whenever a "breathing incident" occurred. My breathing difficulty remained unchanged.

A friend with whom my husband had discussed my hospital visit and problem visited us and shared the issue "THE LAST CHANCE HEALTH REPORT," a health newsletter, Volume 3, Number 5, in which Sam Biser reported his interview with you in the article, "THE TRUE UNKNOWN CAUSE AND CURE OF ASTHMA."

As soon as I finished reading the article I started the water treatment and have been on it since early August. Let me emphasize that I had become very inactive and spoke as little as possible, since activity and speaking caused me breathing difficulty. Within one week of drinking at least eight glasses of water daily, my breathing became easier and less labored. I regained my normal energy. For over three weeks of this date, I have been walking three miles in the morning and three miles in the evening. I did not take the Xanax as I detest tranquilizers, nor have I been on any other medication.

I have since secured your book, "Your Body's Many Cries for Water," read it, and shared it with friends and relatives.

It is my prayer that other people with breathing problems read about you and try the water treatment that has helped me so much.

> *With best wishes!*
> *Sincerely,*
> *Martha Avelar*

☞ ☞ ☞ ☞ ☞

Ms. Paczkowski's letter tells how water helped her overcome her asthma symptoms and also possibly helped improve her eyesight.

Sandra Paczkowski
247 Gedding St
Avoca, PA 18641
May 16, 1997

Asthma/Blindness
Can There Be a Connection?

I have had asthma for three years and have been treated by an allergist and a doctor. Each time I would get a cold (which was frequently), I would also get this horrible cough. Other than the colds and asthma I was perfectly healthy.

Last year, after having a cold and cough, I developed optic neuritis in my left eye which left me with only 20 percent vision in that eye. This year, after having a cold and terrible cough again, I developed optic neuritis in my right eye. You cannot imagine the despair I experienced when this happened because I had been to the best eye hospitals in the East and had been told they could not find a reason for this optic neuritis (they put me through every test imaginable) and they have no cure or operation or any kind of hope for me.

My doctors here treated me with steroids and saved my sight in my right eye. At the same time I was told about the "WATER CURE" for asthma and grabbed at this because it was the only real lifeline I had left. (You have to picture a widow, living alone, not being able to drive or take care of her home, or go to work without begging for help from family and friends. I really thought my life was over.) Immediately I began drinking 64 oz. of water every day and in two days I stopped coughing and have not coughed for five months now or even had a cold, which is a miracle for me.

I am now able to drive, work, cut grass, shovel snow, and go for walks, and, except for the damage done to my left eye, lead a perfectly healthy life. I do see a slight improvement in my eyes and am hoping that if I can stay cough-free for a while, I may get more sight back.

We all think because we drink a lot of coffee, tea, soda or juice that we are getting all the fluids we need, but we don't realize that most of these drinks can dehydrate your body. Water is the most inexpensive, non-invasive, healthy thing we can do for ourselves.

Sincerely,
Sandra Paczkowski

The following letter from Gerald Ward shows how adequate water intake can also cure peptic ulcer disease and stop cravings and addictions, as well as preventing asthma from recurring.

Gerald Wade
PO Box 2009
Florence, AL 35630
August 23, 1993

Dear Sir:

I have been attempting to drink 6-8 glasses of water daily and am pleased to report remarkable results.

My peptic ulcer that bothered me for years has gone into remission. I have been on antacid pills for years too, and now no longer need them—just rarely use one. I no longer take Tagamet and medicines like that.

For years I have had a habit (addiction?) to colas. I am happy to say that I immediately stopped craving them upon starting my water project.

Also, my asthma has diminished noticeably. I am delighted with all the progress I have made just on water.

I am 65 and recently retired and really feeling very good and most certainly intend to continue drinking water as suggested. I am sure there are many other benefits I am receiving from drinking water in quantities like I do now.

It hardly seems enough to just say thanks, but be sure that I am very, very grateful for this revelation.

Best wishes,
Gerald Ward

☞ ☞ ☞ ☞ ☞

In the next letter, you will see how Paul Harvey's discussion of the asthma cure with water in his ABC news program saved a family from disaster.

Christine Warner-Bursian
8225 Elm Drive
Traverse City, MI 49684
June 23, 1995

To Whom It May Interest

I am writing to share my situation with you and offer information that could be helpful to you and those you love and care for.

Three weeks ago my 10 year old son Aaron was diagnosed with allergies (to almost everything but foods!) and asthma. He had suffered most of the fall and winter with nasal congestion, coughing and a constant need to clear his throat. When these symptoms did not respond to traditional treatments our pediatrician referred us to an allergy specialist. The allergist prescribed five different medications/inhalers to use three times per day and gave us a booklet on how we needed to change our lives and our environment. After this appointment, my very active, happy child was upset, scared and depressed. I returned him to school and on my way back I heard the end of a Paul Harvey broadcast about a doctor treating asthma and allergies with water! My initial reaction was skeptical. As I started my son on medications I kept remembering the broadcast. Within two days of beginning medications he felt worse. His mouth and throat burned, the medicine made him irritable, drowsy and sun-sensitive.

At this point I decided to investigate this broadcast further. I called the main office of Paul Harvey News and a very helpful woman looked up the broadcast and gave me the phone number to contact Global Health Solutions. I contacted them immediately and they were also very helpful. I ordered Dr. F.

Batmanghelidj's book "Your Body's Many Cries for Water." I was also given a phone number to call Dr. Batmanghelidj if desired. The book arrived a few days later. I started my son on Dr. Batmanghelidj's recommended re-hydration program with a little added salt and, after less than a week, his symptoms have almost completely stopped and he is feeling great and taking NO medications.

The information and help given us by Dr. Batmanghelidj saved our family much emotional and financial distress that could have gone on for years. Please pass on this information to others. My son was ill and we were distressed by that, but many children actually DIE from this condition every year!

In a Paul Harvey editorial of January 24, 1994 in the Connecticut Post he wrote: "I don't know if Dr. Fereydoon Batmanghelidj's idea is worth anything or not;" also, "Maybe this doctor is just another opportunist selling books, but on the chance that he has something, let's listen..." I can tell you most assuredly that his "idea" is WORTH MUCH! It makes a great deal of sense and is utterly simple and totally effective. I can also attest that he is absolutely not an opportunist selling books. I admit I was skeptical initially. Since my receipt of his book I wrote him a note to thank him, and shortly thereafter I received a personal phone call from him offering help and assistance at any time. He then followed up a few days later to check my son's progress and again offer help. AND HIS PRESCRIPTION WAS WORKING!

Dr. Batmanghelidj has committed himself to get this information to the public in whatever way he can. The medical profession will not listen. He has tried that. It is a terrible crime that so many are suffering when the solution is so simple and readily obtainable. Dr. Batmanghelidj's research and commitment is truly a gift and applies to us all!!

Please help pass on this information to anyone you can. I am committed to doing just that. You are welcome to contact me at any time if you would like.

> *Sincerely,*
> *Christine Warner-Bursian*

☞ ☞ ☞ ☞ ☞

Thank you to Paul Harvey. He has been most supportive on many different occasions and has shared "the water cure" with his dedicated audience.

The following is an e-mail message I received on December 16, 1998 from Mrs. Warner-Bursian, updating me on her son's condition.

My son Aaron is now 13 and a half and has been medication-free ever since I found you! Imagine all these years with five medications if the allergist had had his way! I am eternally grateful to you.

☞ ☞ ☞ ☞ ☞

In Connie Giblin's letter, she shares her experiences with the healing power of water with her own allergies, and explains how promoting "the water cure" is now her full-time job.

Connie Giblin
Box 3298, RD#3
Moscow, PA 18444
May 31, 1996

Dear Dr. Batmanghelidj

As you will recall, I started working for Mr. Bob Butts on January 10, 1996. I was hired to work with him on his "Special Project." This project was to prove to the people of Northeastern Pennsylvania that your Water Program is truly the Greatest Health Discovery in history. Bob said that when we succeed here, then it will sweep the entire country. When I was interviewed on January 4th, I had NO IDEA what I was getting into. Now I know it was the best thing that has ever happened in my life. Your discovery gave me my life back, something I didn't realize I was losing till I started to pay attention to how I was treating my body.

Bob explained your simple solution to gaining good health, that is, drinking two quarts of water daily and implementing a half teaspoon of salt as seasoning in the diet gives most health problems no reason to exist. My desk is only two feet from the water cooler so that was the easy part. Now I had to drink it. I had always drunk water but never really realized what it was doing for me because I was still drinking about two quarts of iced tea a day. That was my biggest downfall. I was dehydrating myself while flooding myself with caffeinated fluids. For every 10-oz glass of tea I drank, I was losing 12 oz of fluids.

I have always suffered terribly with PMS and found that, when I was close to that point, my family would avoid me like the plague. I was irritable, bloated, miserable and very hard to live with. That's putting it mildly to say the least. I also suffered from an eye problem that came about on Memorial Day of 1995.

My eyes got very irritated and itchy. The itchier they got, the more I rubbed them, causing them to blow up and become very red. My eyeballs felt like they had sand in them as well. I went to my doctor three times. Each time I was told I had this or that. I was given three different prescriptions three different times, eye drops, eye cream and pills. Never mind the cost and time involved, but none of these prescriptions worked. The problem came back as soon as I stopped taking or using them. I was just masking the problem.

I was told by a girlfriend about her allergist, so I called and made an appointment. It would have cost $130.00 just to walk in the door before giving my name. Then I would have had to go through an hour of poking with needles to see what I was allergic to. Needless to say, I never went. But I was desperate to find out what the problem was. I have had allergies for most of my life and just thought I was allergic to the state I live in due to the pollen, and I have animals. Boy, was I wrong! After starting on your Water Program and paying attention to my diet, I have never felt better in my life. My energy level has soared. My eye problem has disappeared and my eyes are clearer than they have ever been. My skin is smooth and I have been told my face is glowing!

And you know what means just as much to me? My full-time job is sharing YOUR discovery with people who come into my office and those we meet at the free seminars we give. The joy I see in their faces in such a short time makes me feel like the luckiest person in the world.

Sincerely,
Connie Giblin

☞ ☞ ☞ ☞

Mary Morley's husband, Gene, is another person who discovered the healing power of water in respiratory disease.

F. Batmanghelidj
Foundation for the Simple in Medicine
P.O. Box 3267
Falls Church, VA 22043
September 29, 1997

Dear Dr. Batmanghelidj,

I am so grateful for your book. I heard about Your Body's Many Cries for Water through the Ken Roberts Company. I am writing to you concerning my husband, Gene, 58, who has bronchiectasis. Ever since his many sinus surgeries, starting back in 1984, he has had trouble with his respiratory functions. This past June, he became really sick. He couldn't breathe, was fatigued, and had a constant cough. X-rays were taken and mis-read. Referrals to specialists take time and are not always easy to get in this land of HMOs. Now, in September, Gene finally saw a specialist who said Gene had been walking around with pneu-monia since June. He also broke out in a rash all over his body. I have never seen anything like it--he was covered! Gene has been living on antibiotics for years and now they are not working anymore. The specialist admitted him to hospital for intravenous administration of antibiotics.

This is where you come in, Dr. B. I was reading your book at the time Gene went to hospital, and I started him on the water program while he was in hospital. I am telling you I saw the results within 24 hours. The most noticeable was the cough. Suddenly he wasn't constantly coughing anymore, just once in a while and then it didn't sound so deep in his chest.

It was all uphill from there. I'm sure the antibiotics were helping, but I still think it was the water that brought him around so quickly. He is continuing your program, incorporating the salt as well into his diet.

I mentioned this to the doctor who agreed about the impor-tance of water, but that was the end of it. It's like you said: only if one is on the verge of collapsing from dehydration does one do anything about it. The doctors never considered hydrating Gene, but many, many thanks to you, I did! My hope and intent is to one day have Gene off all medication.

Thank you again.

> Sincerely,
> Mary Morley
> 4615 NW 173rd Place
> Portland, OR 97229

☞ ☞ ☞ ☞ ☞

Dr. Rivera was working at a clinic in Pennsylvania when he wrote me this letter.

Dr F. Batmanghelidj
P.O. Box 3189
Falls Church, VA 22043
October 29, 1993

Dear Dr. Batmanghelidj

Enclosed is a summary of a patient who has been treated with water as part of his therapeutic treatment.

Twelve-year-old male with H/O asthma (non-exertional). Patient has been seen by pediatrician and was put on Proventil inhaler. Patient's mother was given misinformation by pediatrician who stated that, when a crisis arose, to take as many puffs of Proventil until asthma subsides. Because of this misinformation, when patient had next crisis the mother gave patient 6 puffs of Proventil with no amelioration but rather exacerbation of the symptoms of wheezing, chest tightness, lightheadedness and restlessness. The patent was able to lie down but continued to wheeze extensively. The mother gave us a call around 10:30 p.m. with the complaint of wheezing and chest tightness of her son. Immediately we told her to give her son two 8oz glasses of water and a pinch of salt on his tongue. We then told her to call us back in 5 minutes for further instructions. To our surprise, her son had stopped wheezing and his chest tightness had decreased. He was then able to lie down and sleep. The patient has been instructed to continue to drink water and use salt if another attack occurs. The mother has been made aware that, if other medications are needed, to use them as instructed.

Jose A. Rivera, M.D.
Allentown, PA

☞ ☞ ☞ ☞ ☞

Read how water brought an end to Rhonda Stapleton's lifelong attacks of bronchitis and persistent coughing.

Rhonda Stapleton
3423 Oakwood Terrace, NW
Washington, DC 20010
April 17, 1998

Dear Dr. Batmanghelidj,

I suffered from asthma as a small child, which eventually subsided. However, I continued to have debilitating bouts of bronchitis every winter of my life. I cannot remember a single year when I did not have a persistent, hacking cough, starting in the fall and continuing through March. One time this coughing was so violent that I had to be taken to the emergency room. Other times I actually pulled muscles and in one case injured a rib from repeated and violent coughing. Doctors kept prescribing antibiotics, but they had absolutely no effect on the problem, and in fact created other symptoms that just made things worse.

This October I was really dreading what I knew would be six long months of suffering for me and my husband (who is kept awake nights listening to me cough). In my morning contemplation (my religion's form of prayer), I asked to be shown a solution to my problem. Immediately, I heard the word "water," and I knew at once that drinking more water would somehow help me, though I wasn't sure how.

I was never much of a water drinker, so I began to drink more water. I increased my intake to the usual 6-8 glasses a day that doctors usually advise. And amazingly, I had no signs of the bronchitis. But somehow I doubted that the inner guidance I had received was accurate. I began to doubt the correlation between my increased water intake and my improved health. I guess the mind is always looking for facts and figures to back up what the part of us that is divine (soul) already knows.

In any case, just as the period of doubting began, someone at work told me about your book and I ordered it. Your book was the "proof" I was looking for! Your explanation of how dehydration leads to asthma and bronchitis was crystal clear to me, and gave me the renewed determination to keep drinking more water. I also added salt to my diet.

I do not follow your regimen as completely as I would like to. But when I begin slipping, I notice a little congestion in my chest, and I again become attentive to my water intake. I am amazed to report that I have made it through the first winter of my life without any bronchitis, and without the persistent, hacking cough that has troubled me every year of my life.

I am incredibly grateful for your work, and hope you are able to distribute this information in a more global way, as I feel much suffering could be alleviated and many misspent medical dollars saved if only people understood the significance of water to the body's functioning.

> *In heartfelt gratitude,*
> *Rhonda Stapleton*

☞ ☞ ☞ ☞ ☞

Here are some e-mail letters attesting to the benefits of treating asthma and allergies and other problems with water.

Dear Dr. B.

Thank you so much for your book. I've had asthma for nearly forty years and finally experienced marked relief with increased salt and water intake.

> *Thanks again,*
> *Carla Evans*

☞ ☞ ☞ ☞ ☞

Dear Dr. B.

I took Rx antihistamines for 20 years for severe allergies. Since I read your book, I haven't used any for over 3 years now and I am fine. Actually, taking antihistamines or decongestant for a cold will trigger an allergic reaction for me.

My two stepsons live with 5 cats and they formerly had asthma and severe allergies to cats. By the way, the best cure for poison ivy is WATER!

Thanks for your help.

> Sincerely,
> Laura Green

☞ ☞ ☞ ☞ ☞

We passed on the information that you gave on your tape about asthma to a friend who had been to Mexico for a cure and had tried all the drugs for asthma. He usually ends up in the hospital about once a month but the last couple of times he tried the water and salt, his symptoms were relieved rather quickly. Thank you for sharing your knowledge on water.

> Gratefully yours,
> Mary Putters

☞ ☞ ☞ ☞ ☞

Dear Dr. B.

Thank you for your book, Your Body's Many Cries for Water. When my wife introduced me in August 1998, I was a skeptic. For years I had taken antihistamines year round for multiple environmental allergies, along with steroid nose sprays and inhalers for asthma. My two-and-a-half year old daughter had been diagnosed with allergies and asthma and placed on antihistamines and inhalers as well. After reading your book, I and my daughter stopped all our medications. Your presentation on the impor-

tance of water and the dehydrating effects of medications made a lot of sense. I figured, what did we have to lose? We drink water anyway. I didn't have to buy expensive supplements. We could always start up our medications again if it didn't work.

My daughter and I began drinking lots of water with a pinch of sea salt every day. Both my daughter and I removed dairy products from our diet. My daughter's asthma and allergy symptoms immediately went away. My symptoms were greatly reduced and I have seldom used antihistamines since last August.

My wife stopped taking Prozac which she took for depression and trichotillomania (she compulsively plucked her eyebrows until they were hardly there), and began drinking water and adding a pinch of salt a day as well. Within weeks, her eyebrows grew back and her depression has subsided.

> *Sincerely,*
> *Jon Beaty*

🖝 🖝 🖝 🖝 🖝

Dear Dr. Batmanghelidj:

I will write you a formal letter later but I wanted to thank you for your water cure. I have suffered with asthma for the last five years and have tried many natural ways to get rid of it or at least to get improvement. I have needed the inhaler at least two times per day and would wake up wheezing pretty near every morning. I did your cure for two weeks but still drank green tea (I love my caffeine). It did not work. I quit tea last Sunday and the asthma cleared up immediately. I only need the inhaler for hard exercise (ju jutsu class), and I wake up with no wheezing and no need for medication. I even put the water cure on our web site as I am so impressed even at this early time. I know you are onto something. Thank you, and I am telling all of my family.

> *Nick Barry*

🖝 🖝 🖝 🖝 🖝

As you can see, assertions that water is good, water is essential, and you must drink it are not enough. You need to know the reasons you should take water regularly. When you begin to understand the pitfalls of low daily water intake, you will become attentive. What is more, you will begin to realize the many ways your body shows it is short of water, and that this shortage is not always in the same spot or region. In water management, the drought-stricken areas are "rotated." That is why sometimes you manifest dehydration in one area of the body and sometimes in another area.

The next letter is most compelling and instructive. It comes from another medical doctor who had asthma and allergies since childhood.

August 2, 1999

Dear Dr. Batmanghelidj,

I would like to give you my story on how your therapy of drinking water has helped my health. You are free to use this letter as you see fit.

I suffered from a severe case of asthma and allergies my whole life. As a child, I was treated with allergy shots which provided no relief. I found asthma inhalers a constant companion. In fact, I could not be anywhere without an inhaler or risk a severe asthma attack. During this same time I also had a terrible case of allergic rhinitis.

I was miserable during the spring, summer and fall seasons. When I entered medical school, I received some relief of my symptoms from steroid inhalers, both for my lungs and my nasal passages. By using these inhalers throughout the day, I was much more comfortable. But I still found it impossible to be without a daily inhaler for my asthma.

Nowhere in my medical training was it stressed to me the importance of drinking water to control these diseases (or any other conditions). I was thoroughly trained on pharmacology and the "wonders" of drug therapies. Shortly after I finished my residency, I read a review of your book, Your Body's Many Cries for Water. Though I was skeptical your ideas could help me overcome my illness, I decided to get this book.

When I read the book, the simplicity of your hypothesis made complete sense to me. When I realized the coffee and soda that I was drinking was actually leaving me in a dehydrated state, I could begin to understand why I was suffering from asthma and allergies. I immediately began drinking more water and stopped drinking non-water sources.

Within a short time, I began to feel better. My asthma symptoms markedly improved and my allergy symptoms diminished. Though I still had to use my inhalers, I was able to significantly decrease the dosage of medication. I was very pleased with the results, and began recommending this therapy to my patients.

Approximately two years later, I was preparing to give a speech on acupuncture. I decided to tell the audience about the benefits of water, so I read your book again. This time, I noticed the section on the importance of salt. I had almost totally omitted salt from my diet. When I added a pinch of sea salt to my regimen, ALL OF MY SYMPTOMS OF ASTHMA AND ALLERGIES RESOLVED WITHIN TWO DAYS! For the first time in my life, I am now free of all medications and I feel wonderful. Your work has changed my practice and made me a better physician. Thank you.

Sincerely,

David Brownstein, M.D.
Medical Director
Center for Holistic Medicine
5821 West Maple Rd., Suite 192
West Bloomfield, MI 48322

☞ ☞ ☞ ☞ ☞

The next letter, from Roger Wilson in England, shows that water can help the body defend itself against dust mites. Mites are minute members of the spider family. They are transparent and difficult to see with the naked eye. They are parasites and are found on the bodies of animals such as cats, dogs, birds and mice. One variety is classified as "house dust mite." This is the offending agent that often causes a body reaction when it gets into the air passageways and the lungs.

If it is fully hydrated, the body has a most efficient way of defending itself against this parasite—and almost all other parasites that enter the body through the intestinal tract. If the body is in a dehydrated state, its defense systems are shut down, they cannot do a good job of killing all the intruders. Consequently, the body is forced to apply a secondary means of defense. To limit the number of parasites that are airborne and would manage to enter the body and overpower the defense systems, the airways to the lungs begin to shut and make breathing difficult. Roger Wilson's experience and observations highlight the role of water in upgrading the efficiency of the immune systems of the body, in this case against dust mites.

Dear Dr. Batmanghelidj,

My many thanks for your research and wonderful book "WATER."

The commonsense approach to health certainly works. In the past eight weeks I have changed my eating and drinking life style. At 53 it is wonderful to have lost 25 lbs, a lean and fit 6' 181 lbs, and I ran 2.5 miles this morning. Water has played a great part in this transformation, not only the drinking but having a high water content diet.

What is really great is that my dust mite allergy for which I previously took a daily nasal spray has gone—no spray for eight weeks. We even slept without all the special covers on the bed last night!

I can assure you that I will continue to keep your ripple spreading.

Yours,
Roger Wilson

☞ ☞ ☞ ☞

Daphne Sluys found her gluten allergy and other ailments were nothing more than ominous labels for various conditions produced by chronic, unintentional dehydration. Many other people will experience similar relief to Daphne's when they rehydrate their bodies. Her letter follows.

From: Dasmuscle@aol.com
Sent: Thursday, February 03, 2000 2:38 PM
To: DoctorFB@watercure.com
Subject: Thank you.

Dear Dr. Batmanghelidj:

I just found your book "Your Body's Many Cries for Water". It made a big impression on me—like getting hit between the eyes and now I see!

I am 39 and have been chasing symptoms of dehydration most of my life—migraines, joint/growing pains, sinusitis, mild asthma, recurrent pneumonia, chronic tiredness, depression, mysterious allergies (recently diagnosed with gluten intolerance), low thyroid.... I was treated as a hypochondriac by doctors, given Valium as a kid, told I had to live with my sinusitis, told to not eat wheat, lived with migraines after all treatments failed, criticized by family for not "snapping out of my depression and lethargy."

Yet something inside me has kept me looking for the mysterious reason for all these symptoms, which I believed were not normal and which I believed were indicators of distress and therefore not to be "ignored and lived with." You have given me the missing puzzle piece.

I have been struggling to keep my sinuses manageably clear (infection free) by severely limiting gluten in my diet. After 2 days of increased water and salt, my sinuses were 100% clear (wonderful feeling), my breathing was easier (I did not realize how chronically reduced it was) and I have much more energy generally, and my mind is clearer too. Six days and I feel great. Here is the punch line for me—I have been eating wheat these past days. Therefore my gluten intolerance seems to have disappeared with increased water and salt! I am so amazed and excited that I wrote to my naturopath and told her of your book and my experience—she has many patients with the same diagnosis. I am waiting for her response.

My children and my husband are benefitting from more water and salt. In particular my youngest son (6 years old) is much better. I have been chasing the cause of his chronic tiredness, anemia, sinusitis, pneumonia, ear infections for his whole life. His doctor kept telling me "he was just a sick kid, so accept that and move on."

My husband has chronic high blood pressure and had recently been put on a diuretic, which failed to reduce the pressure, so his doctor doubled the dose, without success. He has also been trying to lose weight with "diet products." He is now on more water and salt and his complexion is much better, the whites of his eyes are less bloodshot. No more diet sodas either.

It has only been 6 days so we have a long path ahead, but I am amazed at what I have seen in myself and my family already. I was beginning to think I would acquire some dreadful label like lupus or chronic fatigue syndrome, but instead I have finally found the path to health. It is strange how the Almighty works— I had been praying for guidance to the path to health and went to the bookstore to find a book on lupus, but could not find a decent book, so was walking out when my eye was caught by your book.

I am so excited by the huge impact and consequences of your information that I am telling my friends and family.

I am a licensed massage therapist so get to see clients for various relaxation and medical reasons. Your information is going to make a big appearance in my work. I was especially interested in your chapter on stress and dehydration. Since de-stressing folks is a lot of my business, it is natural for me to direct them to your information. I have contacted the school I trained at because I think we could have really benefitted from your information in our training. I am urging the school (Ashmead College, Washington State) to, at a minimum, include your book on their recommended reading list.

My sister is a physical therapist in South Africa—I directed her to your information too. She tells of many South Africans finding they have better energy when they take salt pills, but that because of the current trend to reduce sodium, the salt pills are difficult to obtain. The heat in South Africa causes a lot of dehydration problems. With your information she will be able to help many people.

Your information is so obvious, yet so brilliant. I shall pray for your continued strength and courage in getting this message to all humanity.

Sincerely,

Daphne Sluys, M.Sc., L.M.P.

(I am embarrassed to admit that I have spent many hours studying anatomy and physiology and never once saw what you saw. Your information is very humbling.) It made a big impression on me—like getting hit between the eyes and now I see!

FAX

Ross Pelton, R.Ph., Ph.D., CCN
4653 Gesner Place
San Diego, CA 92117
Phone: (619)-275-2456
Fax (619)-275-5870 or 275-2456

Date: November 20, 1997
To: Dr. Batmanghelidj
From: Ross Pelton
RE: Water

Dear Dr. Batmanghelidj,

I just wanted to say hello and thank you for your important book about the importance of water.

I ama pharmacist and a certified clinical nutritionist. Since reading your book I have been telling users of steroid inhalers about your book and counseling and educating them about the importance of complete hydration. The results have been astounding. In the past 18 months I have had dozens of patients (or the parents) come back and thank me for having taken the time to discuss this issue with them.

Most of my current professional life is now devoted to being a health educator. I travel around the country teaching nutritional seminars to pharmacists. I specialize in teaching nutrition-related patients counseling skills to pharmacists, and your topic is one of the areas that is always included.

So, this is just a friendly "hello" and a note to let you know that I have picked up your work and am teaching and educating hundreds of pharmacist about this topic around the country.

Keep up the good work.

Healthy regards,

Ross

1 page including cover

Cassandra C. Boughan
805 Adella Avenue
Coronado, CA 92118-2611

Oct. 6, 1996

Dear Dr. Batmanghelidj —

Since I was an infant,
I had been plagued with
chronic allergic and environmental
asthma. I am 35 years old,
and up until 1 year ago, when
my father sent me a copy of
your wonderful book on water,
I was completely dependent
on bronchodialators —.

As a child I took liquid
Marax, as a teenager I took
oral theophylline, and as an

adult I was on a combination
of inhaled steroids and β-agonis·
bronchodilators (Prednisone & Ventolin)
I was worn-out from fighting
for breath, and nervous and

shaky from the medicines' side-effects.

Then, a year ago, I began following the recommendations in your wonderful book. I have not only been asthma-free for over a year now, but am also able to go running without medication, as I do 3-4 times a week.

You have given my life back to me. Bless you and your work.

Sincerely, Cassandra C. Boughan

🖙 🖙 🖙 🖙 🖙

The testimonials you have read speak for themselves. Some of them are from practicing doctors who confirm my clinical and scientific findings.

To show you the seriousness and validity of my scientific views, here is the abstract of my presentation at the 3rd Interscience World Conference on Inflammation, held in Monte Carlo in 1989.

3rd INTERSCIENCE WORLD CONFERENCE ON
INFLAMMATION
ANTIRHEUMATICS, ANALGESICS,
IMMUNOMODULATORS.

ABSTRACT FORM

IMPORTANT: These instructions must be followed completely. Read all instructions before you begin typing on this special form.

Mail to
Scientific Secretariat
3rd Interscience
World Conference
on Inflammation
Istituto di Farmacologia
Via Roma, 55
56100 Pisa (Italy)

Title

Authors

Institute

NEUROTRANSMITTER HISTAMINE : AN ALTERNATIVE VIEW POINT

F. Batmanghelidj, M.D.

Foundation For The Simple In Medicine,

2146 Kings Garden Way, Falls Church, VA. 22043, U.S.A.

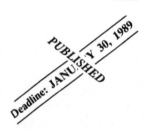

PUBLISHED: JANUARY 30, 1989
Deadline:

ABSTRACT: Advances in histamine research show it to be a neurotransmitter, a neuromodulator and an osmoregulator of the body. While thirst sensation is a failing indicator of now recognized, age-dependent, state of possible cellular and chronic dehydration of the body, to the point that between the ages of twenty to seventy the ratio of the extracellular to the intracellular water content of the body has been shown to change from a figure of 0.8 to almost 1.1, histamine is demonstrating responsibility for the essential osmoregulatory and central dipsogenic functions in the body. Histamine is involved in the initiation of cellular cation exchange, that seems to be supplemental to the role of water in cellular metabolic mechanisms. Histamine is also a modulator of lymphocyte biology and function; through H_1 or H_2 activation of the different lymphocyte subpopulations that have nonrandom distribution of histamine receptors, their functions are integrated. Histaminergic drive for body water regulation and intake brings about the release of vasopressin, which in turn, by possible production of "shower head" cluster perforations of 2 Angstrom units, allowing single file entry of one water molecule at a time through the membrane, promotes increased flow of water through the cell membrane; this function is particularly important for the maintenance of the low viscosity, microtubule directed, microstream flow of the axonal transport system. Vasopressin seem also to act as a modulating cortisone release factor, when constant ACTH secretion can be implicated in the general inhibition of the immune system's functions; histamine may be involved in modulation of neuroendocrine systems, possibly when ACTH feedback mechanism is broken. Next to oxygen water is the single most essential substance for the survival of the body, also recognizing that the dry mouth is not the sole indicator of "free water" deficiency of the body, symptom producing excess histaminergic activity, including chronic pain production, should be judged to be also an indicator of body water metabolism imbalance. The natural primary physiological drives of the histaminergic, the serotonergic neurotransmission (another system involved in the body water regulation, as well as pain threshold alteration) and the angiotensin II for water intake of the body should be acknowledged and satisfied before and during evaluation of the clinical application of antihistamines in treatment procedures, particularly as increased water intake may be the only natural process for the regulation and inhibition of histamine's over production and release. The prolonged use of antihistamines in gastroenterological, psychiatric, seasonal allergic conditions, as analgesics or anti-inflammatory agents without very strict attention to body water intake regulatory functions of the body, by also masking signals of dehydration, may eventually be the cause of cell membrane receptor down-regulation and disturb the integration and balance, and possibly, shift the immune system in an opposite dominant direction and therefore, be responsible for the production of new and continuing change of physiological steady-state situations, incompatible with the total and prolonged well-being of the patient.

Key Words: Histamine, pain, inflammation, immunomodulation, thirst, water

FORMAT FOR ABSTRACT

▼1. Your abstract should be informative, containing: (a) specific objectives; (b) methods; (c) summary of results; (d) conclusions.
2. Single space all typing. Capitalize all letters of the title. The text should be a single paragraph, starting with a 3-space indentation. Leave no top or left margin within the area provided.
3. Abbreviations must be spelled out on first mention, followed by the abbreviation in parentheses.
4. Any special symbol that is not on your typewriter must be drawn in BLACK INK.
5. DO NOT ERASE. Remember that your abstract will appear in a special volume exactly as submitted.
6. Mail first class with 2 photocopies to address given above.
7. If more than one abstract is submitted with the same first author, indicate which abstract should have priority. Other abstracts will have a lower priority.
8. **Please underline speaker's name.**

PUBLISHED; PAGE 37 OF THE ABSTRACT VOL.
3rd Interscience World Conference On Inflammation,
Antirheumatics, Analgesics, Immunomodulators.
Monte-Carlo (Principality Of Monaco), March 15-18, 1989
In Win 89

Point to remember: It is true that all human bodies are absolutely dependent on the regular intake of water and salt, but the internal chemistry of no two persons is identical. The internal chemistry of people with asthma and allergies is obviously outside of the "mainstream" of normal functions, otherwise they would not manifest the outward signs that are labeled as asthma or allergies when they become increasingly dehydrated. In these people, many years of continuous unintentional dehydration have left their slowly establishing chemical imprint that will take some time for reversal and allow the individual's biochemical functions to return to normal.

Unfortunately, some of these people have developed highly reactive allergies to one or other chemical agent, such as to preservatives used in some Chinese foods, to glazing preservatives used in dried fruits, to solvents in beauty products, or, more frequently, to penicillin and other drugs used as medicines.

Among these unfortunate people are some whose allergic reactions are "volcanic" in nature and who very quickly go into bronchial spasm and shock—known as "anaphylactic shock." These people need much longer for their bodies to become less reactive and susceptible to possible suffocation. Although water and salt will help these people in minutes, however, their treatment needs must be in place in seconds. Such persons, who already know and recognize their own "arrow of misfortune" among the offending chemicals, and who are on bronchodialator inhalers, will need to carry their inhalers with them at all times. After a few years of full hydration, and keeping away from their particular allergenic chemicals, their bodies most probably will lose memory of whatever produced the allergic reaction.

The scientific discovery that water has
medicinal properties, it can prevent
diseases, as well as cure them, elevate
the level of our thinking in medicine and
affords us the joy of declaring a natural
end to a vast number of human
diseases in the 21st century.

"I firmly believe that if the entire
materia medica as now used could be
sunk to the bottom of the sea, it would
be all the better for mankind and all
the worse for the fishes."

Oliver Wendell Holmes

6

Lupus

I have for some time been asked for my views and understanding of lupus as a disease. "Can water cure lupus?" is the
question asked of me by many, many people from different parts
of the world.

Since the topic of chronic, unintentional dehydration as a
disease-producing phenomenon in the human body was new, and
I had been confronting an uphill battle for its introduction into
the mainstream of thought in our society, I chose not to engage
in the discussion of lupus at the time. It might have complicated
the process and delayed a satisfactory outcome. Now seems to be
a good opportunity to air my thoughts on the issue. What has
prompted me to take this step is the urgency that was reflected in
the Lupus & Autoimmune Disease Special Issue of *Townsend
Letter for Doctors & Patients*, August/September 1999.

This special issue of the journal contains articles and letters
written by many people, including medical doctors, chiropractors, herbalists, acupressure experts, "philosophers," environ-
mentalists, naturopaths, and patients/authors. The editors of the
journal, who are eminent medical doctors, presented the latest
thoughts on lupus from the perspectives of mainstream and alternative medicine practices.

In all this writing, I did not see any discussion on the importance of water in the prevention or treatment of this disease. This

omission—lack of appreciation for water as a natural medication—got to me, and I started to take a look at lupus as a complex of conditions produced by dehydration, which is my perspective of the origin of painful degenerative disease of the human body.

One of the editors, Alan R. Gaby, M.D., began his editorial with a remark that was, in my opinion, the most insightful statement on lupus in all of the journal's presentations. He wrote: *"The conventional view of autoimmune disease is that the immune system, for no good reason at all, goes awry and attacks the body's own tissues. But, considering the intimate connections that exist between the mind, the brain and the immune system, it might be pretentious to assume that the human system has no good reason for doing what it does. Perhaps it has a reason that we don't understand."*

In this section, I will try to show that we are the problem. We absolutely don't understand the human body. The human body has very sound physiology-based reasons for doing what it does, including the manifestation of various symptoms that we have categorized as diseases.

In my researched opinion, chronic, unintentional dehydration can rear its ugly head in many different ways. Not recognizing persistent water shortage inside the cells of the body as a symptom-producing state of physiology—in the fourth dimension of time—we in medicine have grouped and labeled different concurrently occurring outcomes of various regional or local "droughts" as separate conditions. Naturally, since without water nothing lives, and comparative dehydration puts the body on its pathway to death, the more distinct and severe the multitude of manifestations that should be recognized as products and complications of drought, the closer would be the life-journey's end.

In my view, one such conglomerate of conditions has been grouped under the label of "systemic lupus erythematosis," SLE or *lupus* for short.

In this chapter, I will identify the various markers of SLE and explain why I think simple "water deficiency" is the root of the problem. Before I do this, we need to have an idea of what lupus is considered to be.

What Is Lupus?

Lupus has until now been classified as a "disease of unknown etiology." Etiology means cause or reason for existence.

- It is a chronic disease that involves several organ systems.

- It is classified as an autoimmune disease, a condition where the immune system attacks some of the body's own tissues.

- It is a condition where the body produces a wide array of antibodies against its own tissues. Some antibodies attack the nucleus of the cell, some attack the membranes on or inside the cells; others attack the blood proteins, the structures inside the cells, and more. The tissues most affected are the blood vessels in the kidneys, the lungs, the brain, the skin, and the joints. When blood vessels are attacked, swelling, redness and even bleeding in the tissues can occur. The process is called *vasculitis*.

- It is a condition that in 1948 was discovered by a researcher, Hargraves, to have particular types of cells called LE cells. LE cells are white cells that have quickly and successively "ingested" other cells. They characteristically reveal in their interior a number of undigested nuclei from the ingested cells.

- Today, because of advances in blood testing techniques, diagnosis of lupus rests mainly on identifying various autoimmune antibodies that can be seen when a person also presents other clinical symptoms and signs. LE cells may not necessarily be present, but as long as the blood picture indicates it, the label of lupus is attached to the patient.

- Diagnosis of lupus is based on clinical symptoms, and on blood and skin tests. Some 70 to 80 percent of the people who are diagnosed as having lupus show LE cells, 95 to 100 percent show antibodies to the structure of the nucleus in the cell, and 70 percent show antibodies to the DNA structure itself.

According to a 1994 survey by the Lupus Foundation of America, SLE affects between 1.4 and 2 million Americans. The ratio of women to men affected by SLE is around 9:1. In some reports, the figures are as high as 19:1. Women are affected early in life, and African-Americans and Latinos are affected more than other races. The actual pathology of the disease is the same in all ages, but children tend to show more symptoms in their kidneys. In older people, the disease is less progressive. Lupus in children affects boys and girls equally. Drug-induced lupus affects men and women equally.

Before cortisone was introduced as a treatment, life expectancy of the afflicted was merely a few years. Now, with cortisone treatment and lifestyle adaptation, life expectancy has been significantly prolonged. The label of lupus by itself can shorten life due to fear of the disease. The reason is that fear, anxiety and emotional stress bring about a pattern of hormonal and chemical secretions that put the body on the pathway of lowered resistance and susceptibility to infections and disease.

The diagnosis of lupus is based on clinical manifestations of any three of the following conditions, plus the appropriate blood tests confirming the disease:

- Extreme tiredness

- Persistent headaches

- Skin rashes on the bridge of the nose and under the eyes. About 80 to 85 percent of lupus patients present this "butterfly rash" on the nose and two sides of the face. At an earlier pre-rash stage, the skin can for some time be "flushed" (known as "malar flush") before it develops a fully blown rash.

- Presence of LE cells

- Muscle and joint pains

- Diffuse or patchy hair loss

- Psychiatric manifestations, seizures, psychosis and organic brain damage—loss of speech, loss of memory, loss of nerve function such as difficulty in swallowing, or excessively painful sensations. Even a gentle wind current can cause pain.

- Kidney damage—blood in the urine, loss of too much protein in the urine (milky urine), inability to get rid of urea, "hypertension of renal origin"

- Pain in the chest or abdomen caused by inflammation of membranes covering the organs and the intestines

- Coldness of the extremities—Raynaud's disease

- Photosensitivity

- Disc-like eruptions and swellings of the skin—discoid lupus

- Persistent and recurring ulcerations in the mouth and on the mucosa inside the nose

Lupus: The Survival Strategy of a Drought-Stricken Body

Let us look at all the symptoms that result in a diagnosis of lupus, and see how easily they can be explained from the vantage point of our understanding of dehydration. We will then look at the connection between simple water shortage in the body and the blood tests that are the telltale indicators of what the body does when it is short of water and the raw materials that water carries to the various parts of the body.

Tiredness and Fatigue: The incorrect assumption that all beverages function in the body in the same way as simple water is fundamental to persistent dehydration. As has been explained, dry mouth is not an accurate indicator of water shortage in the body. The body can suffer from dehydration before presenting dry mouth as a sign. Add to this problem the wrong choice of fluids that dehydrate the body even more when your urge to drink surfaces, and you have a crisis on your hands.

The brain receives its bulk of energy from water. Hydroelectric energy is generated by the rush of water through the cell membranes exactly where energy is needed for cell-talk among the 9 trillion cells of the nervous system and their connections to the muscles and joints. Another process of energy transfer from water is called hydrolysis. Water energizes the breakdown of materials such as starch, proteins and fats to their final chemical byproducts that are then used as fuel by the brain cells. In dehydration, this process is inadequate and the brain suffers from a low-energy state that we have labeled as tiredness or fatigue. The more dehydrated the body, the more fatigued it becomes.

To explain how water generates energy when it is involved in chemical reactions, the energy formula for hydrolysis of one of the "energy blocks," magnesium ATP (ATP—adenosine triphosphate,) calculated by P. George and co-workers and published in 1970, is presented below. Magnesium ATP has 600 units of energy stored in it. When it is hydrolyzed, the energy value in its components increases about 10 times to 6,435 units of energy.

In Living Cells,
Water is the Primary Source of Energy

$$MgATP^{2-} + H_2O = ADP^{3-}/ADPH^{2-} + Mg^{2+}/H^+ + H_2PO^{4-}/HPO_4^{2-}$$

600   **1500**   **600**   **998**   **1168**   **318**   **1251**

The units of energy are measured in **Kilojoules**
(Energy required to raise the temperature of one pound
of water through one degree Fahrenheit = one Joule)

Apply this equation to the total body functions that depend on the energy-generating property of water, and you will realize why dehydrated people are low in energy. You will realize why water, not coffee, is the best "pick-me-up" you can find. Caffeine indiscriminately causes different parts of the nervous system to lower the threshold of energy release from their vital reserves. They use up their precious energy, which is stored for crisis management, on trivial pursuits. This is the reason the body shows lassitude after a few cups of coffee.

Persistent Headaches: The brain has priority over the rest of the body for delivery of water and the raw materials that are transported in water. The brain is 2 percent of the total body weight but is allocated 20 percent of the total circulation of the body. When the body is dehydrated, the brain is highly stressed, even though we do not realize it. The brain is a 'silent brooder!" It has to deal with its normal routine of "mind-brain-environment-body" coordination, as well as dealing with a fair and just allocation of the available water and raw materials to the rest of the body according to each organ's priority of function.

To do its work, the brain needs to receive more of the blood flow to "pump" some of its water into its own fluid environment and to get rid of its toxic waste. Expanding circulation to the brain tissue is controlled by the neurotransmitter histamine and its subordinate regulators. The brain capillaries are well endowed with type-2 histamine receptors (H2 receptors). When stimulated, H2 receptors dilate the brain capillaries. Histamine and its subordinate regulators signify their engagement by causing pain.

Pain means dehydration. The conscious mind should understand this, but our inaccurate education about the human body shows this understanding is lacking from our pool of knowledge.

Butterfly Rash: The typical rash of lupus is normally on the bridge of the nose, extending onto the cheeks. It resembles a butterfly perched on the nose (Figure 10). Initially, there is a "malar flush" that can change to scaly skin eruptions and red, round, and somewhat flat, spots. In some people, the rash can be more wide-spread and extend to the forehead, the chin and around the lips.

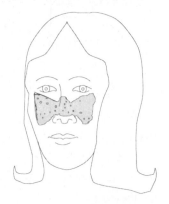

Figure 10

Why Is Malar Flush a Feature in Dehydration of the Body?

The design and nature of the face is not only to house the eyes, the nose and the mouth. It is made with other functions in mind. It is a sensory center that houses the organs of sight, sound, smell and taste. These are the senses we are aware of, but the face has other sensory capabilities that we have not yet studied fully and do not yet understand their mechanisms. Nonetheless, these additional sensory capabilities do exist and we should gradually incorporate this fact into our appreciation of the importance of our face. It must be appreciated for more than just its looks.

The human face is also a "receptor dish" for "waves of energy" that do not achieve the intensity of light. These "infrared" ranges of radiating energy carry with them information that the human body needs to incorporate in its routine evaluation of its environment and whatever knowledge that can be assimilated from that "experience." This activity is a part and an extension of the nervous system and takes priority over other functions of the body.

Animals use this faculty extensively when they hunt in the dark. A particular species of desert mouse is totally blind; it has no eyes and lives under the sand. It zeroes in on similarly sub-sand-dwelling prey, using the mechanism for eyeless "seeing" described below. There are other animal species that use this "extrasensory" perception for guidance.

This same type of "sight" occurs in humans. If you watch blind people walking along a road or sidewalk, you will notice that they constantly turn their heads from one side to another, as if detecting objects in their way. In fact, they are scanning their path of movement. They seem to become aware of obstacles before knocking into them. I am told that even with 100 percent loss of vision, the blind do still have some "sight." This statement achieved validity for me when I read about a German boy who is blind but rides his bicycle in the midst of downtown traffic in one of the heavily populated cities in Germany, and the Russian girl who moves around with agility and speed, negotiating flight of stairs, even though totally blind.

How Is It Possible to "See" Without Eyes?

To learn more about the simple explanation I am about to give, you need to read Chapter 4 of *The Blind Watchmaker,* by Richard Dawkins. One of the most outstanding scientists of our times, he is a distinguished biologist at Oxford University in England. BBC Television has serialized his information in a number of documentary programs.

Professor Dawkins makes a simple statement in his book: there exists a Creator. The analogy he uses is simple. A watch is invented by man and has many tiny pieces that, when assembled according to the watch's design, become a measuring instrument for the transition of time. The argument used is: if you reduce a watch to its individual components and then put the pieces in a spinning machine and spin them N number of times, the pieces will never become a watch again by "random selection" of the "spin-positioned" components. You need intelligence and a pair of hands to put the pieces together in the order that the designer had intended.

Professor Dawkins sets out to explain evolution as a step-by-step process of creation, all the time improving on the previous stages and designs. I will not get into the detail of evolution and creation here, but would like to use the source of information that defines the evolution of various light-sensitive anatomical parts until the formation of the eye as we know it. There seem to exist lensless light-sensitive patches, cups, holes or pits within the lower levels of the animal kingdom. Photosensitive pits register information, but are not designed to focus a sharp image. The species concerned use these "photosensitive pits" to the limit of what they need.

Since photosensitive pits are anatomical realities in living species, it should not be considered far-fetched to assume that we humans also employ this technology as a supplement to our visual apparatus. Photosensitive pits—or more likely, "patches"—are a part of our visual apparatus. They expand our capability to monitor our environment, and are located mainly on our faces.

What provides additional support to this concept is the size and placement of the fifth nerve of the brain itself—the trigeminal nerve. We have two of them, one on each side of the brain. Their branches enter the space behind the skin of the face from three different locations, above the eyes, below the eyes, and the lower chin. These nerves are much thicker than the ordinary nerves that reach the skin in other parts of the body. Their thickness in proportion to their surface area of service indicates that the trigeminal nerves, which supply the face and the forehead only, are engaged in more complicated work than just dealing with the sensation of heat, cold and touch.

In order to perform their function of transmission of information in the nerve system, the skin receptors of the trigeminal nerve depend absolutely on the availability of adequate water. In dehydration, the regular circulation to the skin surfaces is shut down to prevent water loss through evaporation from the skin surface. However, increasing circulation to the vicinity of these nerves of the face becomes of paramount importance, hence the formation of the malar flush. Later, the nerve endings demand even greater circulation to get more water to clear their toxic waste.

This program of increased vascularity to nerve fibers and their receptors is normally under the control of histamine. It is interesting to note that there are between 7,225 and 12,100 histamine-producing mast cells per cubic centimeter of skin. (The original reference stated per cubic millimeter, but I think there is an error in this documentation.) Thus, the skin is well endowed with the source of histamine to organize the "inflammatory" process in the vicinity of the nerves, hence the skin eruptions on the faces of symptom-producing dehydrated individuals who suffer from lupus.

It is a fact that the human body can decipher information from natural wavelengths of energy that do not achieve light-band intensity. According to Nick Begich, M.D., electromagnetic-energy force recognition by the human body is now the subject of extensive research by military forces for its possible military application. The research is directed at a means of *pulsing, shaping* and *focusing* the energy in a way that it could couple with the body and take over the natural physiological functions such as sleeping, emotional interpretations, voluntary muscle movements, memory obliteration, or memory replacement. The purpose of this research is its possibility of crowd management.

Dr. Begich and I were presenting talks at the Annual Convention of the World Foundation for Natural Science in Lindau, Germany, in October 1999. Dr. Begich is an internationally recognized authority in his field and his presentations are based on thousands of documents he has reviewed. He is of the opinion that "pulsed-energy technology" is advanced to the point of its already having been employed in some situations. He thinks one such occasion was the Gulf War. It seems that Saddam Hussein's Republican Guards were the target of pulsed-energy mind control by the US Air Force. Their volition to fight was wiped out and instead they were programmed to surrender. That is the reason they did not fire a shot, but surrendered in their tens of thousands, and the allies did not suffer casualties.

This type of technology has its advantages and also has a serious downside. The downside is that the people become puppets in the hands of their government. Any politician who gets access to the means of delivering his/her "message" to the public in elections will have an unfair advantage over other candidates. This is how freedoms could be lost and dictatorial states could become established.

George Orwell predicted the Big Brother takeover of the world in his book, *1984*. It seems the technology to do just that is now in the hands of our government and its "big money" manipulators. If you wish to read works by Dr. Begich, call Earthpulse Press 907-249-9111, or go to his Website, www.earthpulse.com.

I went into this amount of detail to explain a simple rash on the face so that I could at the same time introduce you to a new understanding of your face, and explain why water is essential to maintain the integrity of what your face has to do.

Lupus Erythematosis Cells

What is an LE cell? It is a large white cell, or macrophage, that has devoured a number of damaged cells and has not had time to digest their contents. We need to realize that the human body has a sophisticated recycling program and utilizes even the last molecule of a useful ingredient. Naturally, the process involves the "execution" of inefficient and dying cells—or transformed aggressive cells that could grow to a fully blown cancer—and the "carnivorous" digestion of their bodies by mobile executioners. But this does not happen willy nilly. There is a system involved.

The system is simple. When a cell does not receive an adequate supply of its needed raw materials for use as energy and its manufacturing processes, it taps into its own energy reserves—very much like during hard times when one depletes one's savings and has to rely on food stamps. In the body there is no such things as "food stamps," "overdrafts," or "family loans." The system imposes a strict rationing program. Less-capable cells are sacrificed and their immediately useful contents are shared with their neighbors—strictly "cannibalism."

The mechanism is again simple. There are certain types of antibodies secreted by roving white cells that are capable of puncturing holes in the membrane of the cells that must die and spilling the doomed cells' fluid content into their immediate environment. The solid components remain in the interior of the compromised membrane. In the spilled fluids from the "killing fields" there is much loose calcium—spent fuel or ash—that is a sign of overspent energy. This environmental overload of calcium activates the transglutaminase enzyme system.

Among the many significant roles of this enzyme is the mummification and hardening of the cell membrane. The process is called *apoptosis*. The mummified cells are recognized and swallowed one after another by the scavenging macrophage cells, until the macrophage cells acquire many hard-to-digest cell remains.

If cars park in a no parking area, the police put a sticker on the windshield of the offending cars. Tow trucks are called and the cars are removed from the no-park zone.

Very much like the sticker on cars to be towed, the apoptotic cells carry a protein marker on their membranes that invite the cannibalistic cells to consume the mummified cells. Laden with the bodies of the consumed cells, the cannibalistic cells are assumed to be the typical LE cell. It seems the purpose of this process is to reduce the population of cells that cannot be adequately supplied with water and nutrients, to immediately recycle their locally usable component, and to carry away the carcasses of the killed cells for further transformation. In essence, this process is repeated continuously when lupus is in its active state.

It is my view that unless this process of "depopulation" is efficient, dehydration and inefficient delivery of primary material will cause certain cells to transform into their earlier primitive forms. Primitive cells possess aggressive, "selfish" genes that take over the cell activity and overgrow their boundaries and form cancerous growths that can thrive in an oxygen-depleted environment. In other words, lupus is the more life-supportive program of dehydration physiology of the body than the alternative of cancer formation. What determines which direction the body goes is determined by the mind-body-environment-lifestyle connections. I will discuss this connection more fully in my next book, *ABC of Cancer and Depression*.

Dehydration: The Mind-Body-Immune-System Connection

I need to get a little technical in this segment. I need to explain the relationship of dehydration to the immune system upheaval at the level necessary for researchers and medical professionals to see the science behind my thoughts and words.

The brain is 85 percent water. Comparative dehydration of the brain cells causes them the silent anxiety of drying up. It is most stressful. At the same time, the brain has to deal with lots of cell-talk to maintain "mind-brain-environment-body" activity and coordination. The brain needs water to energize its delicate functions.

In dehydration and "emotional stress," the brain takes pre-emptive actions to bring along more water and raw materials for

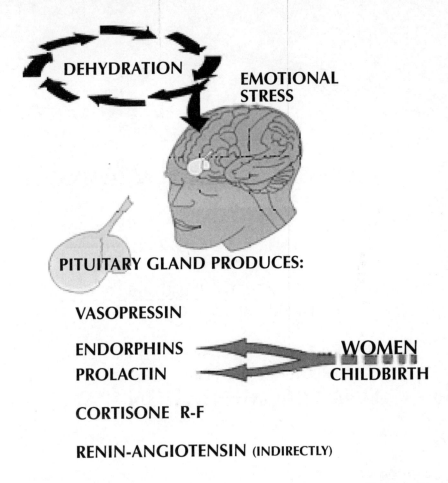

Figure 11

its own needs. It manufactures a number of hormones and transmitters to coordinate this activity (Figure 11). The brain's course of action is coordinated through secretions of the pituitary gland. The "hormone/transmitters" that are secreted include vasopressin, endorphins, prolactin, cortisone release factor, and renin-angiotensin.

Vasopressin is a hormone that converts its counterpart receptor into a hollowed container with a cluster of tiny perforations. These perforations are designed to filter only water out of the serum and to let one water molecule pass through the holes

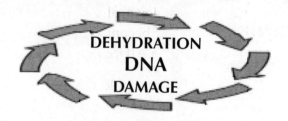

INCREASED CORTISONE ACTIVITY

- CAUSES **INTERLEUKIN-1** ACTIVITY AND DEPRESSES **INTERLEUKIN-2** ACTIVITY

- **ILK-2** STIMULATES THE IMMUNE SYSTEM AND INTERFERON PRODUCTION

- **ILK-1** INHIBITS THE IMMUNE SYSTEM AND IS INDIRECTLY RESPONSIBLE FOR **DNA FRAGMENTATION**

Figure 12

into the cell—much like a showerhead. Vasopressin is at the same time a very strong cortisone releaser. It is a cortisone release factor (CRF). Apart from vasopressin, the pituitary gland also secretes another distinct CRF. In this way, the body chemistry of a dehydrated person becomes influenced by two kinds of very strong CRF secretions.

CRF stimulates some white cells to secrete a substance called interleukin-1 (IL-1). At the same time, these potent cortisone-releasing agents strongly inhibit two other chemicals that would otherwise neutralize the impact of IL-1. These are interleukin-2 and interferon—Figure 12. Histamine, the primary water regulator, strongly, and simultaneously to the action of CRF, inhibits the production and release of interleukin-2 and interferon in the body. Thus, in dehydration, two agents engaged in the drought management programs of the body shut down the defense side of the immune system. The shutdown of IL-2 and interferon production is the reason the body becomes vulnerable to bacterial and viral infections—such as in AIDS.

When IL-1 achieves an appreciable presence in the circulation, it stimulates further secretion of CRF. In this way, as long as dehydration/stress engages the brain cells' activity, the vicious cycle of IL-1 production will continue. (See Figure 13.)

At a certain juncture in the chemical pathways, substances such as interleukin-6 are secreted. IL-6 can destroy the nuclei of the insulin-producing cells of the pancreas. The reason the

Biochemical Pathways of Autoimmune Diseases

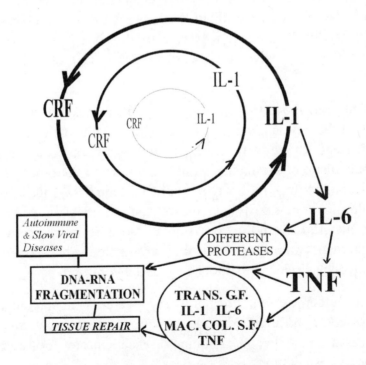

Key words : IL-1= interleukin-1: IL-6 = interleukin-6 :
TNF = tumor necrosis factor : CRF = cortisone release factor :
TRNS.G.F. = transforming growth factor :
MAC.COL.S.F. = macrophage colony stimulating factor.

Figure 13

insulin-producing cells are not destroyed in everyone that becomes persistently dehydrated is because there exists a mechanism that makes these cells dormant and inactive when the body is short of water.

Other chemicals produced for similar outcomes include tumor necrosis factor (TNF), transforming growth factor (TGF), and macrophage colony stimulating factor (MCSF). They eventually cause "randomly selected" tissue breakdown and damage, followed by remodeling of the damaged site. The purpose of the initial breakdown is to recycle some primary raw materials that the brain/body needs. Topping the list of urgently needed primary materials is the water that is held inside the cells.

The delicate control system for the secretion of these hormones depends on a type of feedback mechanism that is installed in the cell membrane of the secretory cells, as well as some cells in a special part of the brain. These cells constantly monitor the blood level of the activators of tissue breakdown. The efficiency of the feedback system in these cells depends on the level of water that is available in between their two-layered cell membrane.

If the cell is well hydrated, the feedback mechanism is efficient. If the cell is dehydrated, the feedback mechanism is inefficient and the chemical-manufacturing process engaged in "cannibalistic crisis management" continues to the point of getting out of control. In this type of process, the CRF and IL-1 that should only temporarily become engaged in releasing some primary materials from the body's own tissues get stuck on the job and "remain commissioned"—their production is not stopped by their feedback mechanism because of dehydration.

The outcome of one form of this type of crisis management of a stressed/dehydrated body that has to resort to cannibalism of its own tissues is called autoimmune disease. One form of autoimmune disease is lupus.

F. Tjernstrom and associates have published the results of

important research in the *Journal of Lupus,* #8, 1999, pages 103-108. The research shows that IL-1 activity is strongly implicated in lupus disease. Those with constant IL-1 activity in their bodies are 700 percent more likely to suffer from lupus than those without IL-1 activity.

The antihistamine activity of water and salt is essential to arrest this vicious cycle of events that breaks down the body's own tissues under the direction of interleukin-1. Water and salt inhibit histamine activity and allow the release and activity of interleukin-2 and interferon to neutralize the action of interleukin-1. Thus, water and salt are vital medications in the treatment of lupus.

In addition to water and salt, a balanced diet, initially high in sugar and carbohydrates to promote insulin secretion by the body, is vital to assist in the reversal of "cannibalistic biochemistry"—catabolism—of the body. Insulin converts the biochemical trends in the body into tissue buildup rather than breakdown. After the initial introduction of more sugar in the diet, food intake has to be high in essential amino acids, essential fatty acids, green vegetables, fruits, vitamins and minerals. For more information, see Chapter 8.

Vasculitis in Lupus

Three different kinds of cells are heavily endowed with histamine-producing capabilities: some brain cells, basophil lymphocytes, and mast cells.

The basophils and mast cells also manufacture heparin, a chemical that "thins" the blood and prevents it from clotting, and platelet activating factor, a chemical that activates the platelets that normally cause the blood to clot.

Why do you think the mast cells or basophils possess two contradicting enzymes and secrete them at the same time? One prevents clotting and the other activates platelets that promote clotting. The reason is simple if you look at the philosophy of water circulation.

When platelets are activated, they secrete the serotonin that they have collected and stored. Serotonin under special circumstances causes increased vascular permeability in very small blood vessels—it can even cause gaps or "surgical slits" in the capillaries—while it constricts large vessels and raises the pressure in the arterial system (*Serotonin and Microcirculation*, Karger 1986; ISBN3-8055-4163-5). The serum (the fluid component of blood minus its blood cells), or even the whole blood, gushes out through the gaps, but does not clot because of the heparin. The red cells—virtual water bags—that also get out of the blood vessels break down and spill their contents in the area that is desperately in need of water. The solid waste from the blood is dealt with later.

Blood is almost 94 percent water; the red cells also consist of mostly water with "hemoglobin coloring." When the system dumps two pints of blood into the intestine or as it bleeds into the tissues, 94 percent of that volume—water—goes immediately back into the circulation, and the solid waste is dealt with as a secondary process.

The rationale of this type of bleeding in the kidneys and the lungs is that both of these organs need lots of "free water" to do their job efficiently. Getting it this way is the only logical process when the body is already dehydrated and no fresh water is coming in.

This process of bleeding takes place in the lungs and kidneys on a microscopic scale. It is identified as a distinct condition called "pulmonary-renal syndrome." The same process is also seen in lupus. It also takes place in the intestinal tract on a larger scale and more frequently. Labels of gastritis, duodenitis or colitis are attached to localized, dehydration-produced vasculitis of the intestinal tract.

I recognized this phenomenon when I treated over 3,000 cases of peptic ulcer disease with water—many patients had bleeding ulcers. I researched the mechanism some time later. In bleeding ulcers, a great deal of blood is dumped in the intestinal tract and its water is reabsorbed to avert overconcentration of the blood and a subsequent catastrophic complication of widespread clotting in the brain and elsewhere. When the process takes place under the skin, it is called a purpura.

A less drastic and more frequently seen alternative to bleeding is to commence a water preservation program and shut down one or other system—hence asthma in children or drastic reduction of urine volume to the point of producing orange-colored urine in older people. These conditions are complications of chronic, unintentional dehydration.

Muscle and Joint Pains

Pain in the body, unless it is from infection or injury, is a sign of dehydration in the area where pain is felt. In a physically active part of the body that does not receive adequate water to supply it with the necessary raw materials and to wash away the toxic waste of metabolism, acidity will increase and at a certain point the nerve endings of the area will pass the information to the brain. The brain, or "conscious mind," registers this chemical environmental change as pain.

Normally, uninjured muscles reflect pain on two counts. One is the buildup of lactic acid in muscle tissue that is overused when it is dehydrated and the acid and toxic waste of muscle metabolism cannot be washed away. The other reason is the fact that muscle tissue is freely sacrificed when the body is feeding on itself. The process is called "gluco-neo-genesis," meaning remaking of sugar from the body's reserves and its own structures.

Cortisone activity, prodded by CRF, is instrumental in dismembering the muscle structure. On a larger scale, this very painful process is often called "muscular dystrophy."

Lupus and Mind-Brain Involvement

When each molecule of myoglobin of the muscle tissue is dismembered, four chemical hooks, called *pyrrole rings*, that grip onto one unit of iron are broken loose and excreted from the body. Unfortunately, each pyrrole unit, before its excretion, hooks onto one molecule of zinc and one unit of vitamin B6 and pulls them out of the body too. Thus, dehydration—in the fourth dimension of time—and its consequential and continuous breakdown of muscle tissue can result in zinc and vitamin B6 deficiency. Vitamin B6 and zinc are vital for brain cell activity. They are essential for the production of neurotransmitters in the brain.

Excess pyrrole excretion is recognized as being associated with neurological and disperceptive disorders of the mind. Another factor in mental disorders is excess histamine activity of the body coupled with copper deficiency. (*Nutrition and Mental Illness* by Carl C. Pfeiffer, Ph.D., M.D., ISBN 0-89281-226-5).

Another unfortunate consequence of dehydration is the excessive use of two essential amino acids by the liver to neutralize toxic waste that cannot be cleared out of the body. These amino acids are tryptophan and tyrosine, which are normally used by the brain cells to be converted to neurotransmitters. Tryptophan is normally converted by the brain into serotonin, melatonin, tryptamine and other brain-active components.

In depression and serious emotional problems, there is a serotonin deficiency in the brain—this is the rationale for the use of Prozac, which slows the destruction of the available serotonin in the body. Naturally, if the neurotransmitter shortages are in the sensory side of the brain, the outcome is sensory neurological problems. If the deficiency of the primary materials is located on the motor side of the brain, the consequence is "irregular and uncoordinated movements" of the body. The organs that are most used are more prone to become deficient first, hence irregular movements of the hands, face, chewing and swallowing, and so on.

Photosensitivity in Lupus

The tryptophan content of the eye is vital to its function. According to Seymour Zigman of the Department of Ophthalmology, University of Rochester School of Medicine, New York (*Progress in Tryptophan and Serotonin Research*, de Gruyter, pages 449-467), the filtering pigments that protect the lens and retina of the eye in animals are tryptophan oxidation products. The pigments derived from tryptophan are vital to light filtration. Naturally, tryptophan deficiency, brought about by persistent dehydration, leaves the eyes vulnerable and unprotected in intense light. This is my understanding of the cause of photosensitivity in lupus.

Raynaud's Phenomenon

The roughly 100 trillion cells of the body are indisputably dependent on water for their survival and efficiency of function. The water-dependent body needs a certain amount of "fresh" and "unmixed" water for its daily functions. If you give it less than the amount of pure water that it needs, it begins to take precautionary water-conservation measures. It begins to shut down certain comparatively unimportant functions. It is forced to do so. It has no alternative.

One of these conservation measures is heat preservation when the body is exposed to a cold environment. As you now realize, water is the primary source of energy in the body. A component of the heat-preservation measures in dehydration is an integrated shutdown of the circulation to the skin. The extremities are easier to control than the trunk of the body, hence a dehydrated person will experience cold hands, feet, nose, and ears. It is my understanding that Raynaud's phenomenon of cold and "blue" extremities is the body's crisis heat-conservation procedure associated with its drought management programs.

Lupus: A Conglomeration of Dehydration-Produced Disorders

From my scientific perspective, lupus is a label put on a basket of conditions that are produced by persistent dehydration of the body. I can even add more labels, such as muscular dystrophy, multiple sclerosis and others, to the list.

From the vantage point of research of the molecular outcome of dehydration, we can put a new logical perspective to what the body does for its drought management that we never understood before. We labeled its telltale markers as this or that disease. Lupus is one such label.

Dr. A. Coutinho, of Gulbankian Science Institute in Portugal, after attending the 5th International Lupus Conference, expressed his views and evaluated lupus research in an article published in the *Journal of Lupus,* #8, 1999, pages 171-173. "Obviously, since the established frameworks and prevalent ideas feed forward on themselves, it will always be easier to add some more of the same to the dominant views than to fight the establishment with something new.... It follows that leaving behind preconceived ideas on tolerance and autoreactivity will certainly help, but a novel idea for the general principles of the disease process would be even better."

Well, Dr. Coutinho, please take a look at chronic unintentional dehydration as a topic in the research of lupus. As I have tried to explain, the answers might fall into place infinitely more quickly than may be imagined.

7

New Way of Resuscitating Drowning Victims

I am introducing this section in the book to share a new way of dealing with drowning victims. It is in contrast to the conventional way where we immediately try to perform CPR on a person whose lungs are full of water so that the air we try to push in has no means of getting into the water-logged lungs. The air we blow into the lungs is not able to replace the water that is filling the alveoli. We first must drain the water out of the lungs before oxygen can enter the lungs and get into the bloodstream. My new method shows how this should be done.

I first learned this simple, commonsense way of immediate help for a drowning victim when my younger brother was fished out of our home pool. He was no more than four and I was about 11 years old. There were eight of us playing in the garden of our house. We never noticed that Dariush was missing until his nurse realized he was not among us. She looked around and called his name. When there was no response, we all became concerned and started searching. That was when the cook noticed his half-submerged body floating face down in the pool. He was pulled out of the water and the telltale blue color of his body and his locked jaws told the whole story: he had stopped breathing. When the nurse saw his color and no sign of life in his body, she started lamenting and howling with such intensity that everyone in the house and on the street came to see what had happened.

Luckily, my father was at home and he ran to see who was hurt. His amazing intelligence took over as soon as he saw Dariush had drowned. He told the cook, who was holding Dariush's lifeless body in his arms, to hold him by the legs and turn him upside down. My father worked his fingers into Dariush's mouth and pulled his locked jaws apart. As soon as Dariush's mouth was forced open, almost half a bucket of water poured out of his mouth. In this way, Dariush's lungs were cleared of their water content. My father smacked Dariush a couple of times on his back. He then told the cook to hold Dariush upside down on his (the cook's) back and run around the yard. By the time the cook returned with Dariush, my brother had begun breathing and had started to cry.

This simple maneuver saved Dariush's life. Years later, I successfully tested it a second time when a college student was pulled out of the water at my sports club's pool. She had been missing from the group of college students who had taken over the pool for their sports hour. They must have thought she had gone to the restroom. Only when they noticed someone at the bottom of the deep end of the pool, did their instructor realize what had happened. I was passing by and heard the commotion. I arrived as the girl was being taken out of the water. She, too, was blue and had stopped breathing. I got the club doorman to hold her upside down and I forced her mouth open. Lots of water flowed out of her mouth. In her case, I chose to resuscitate her by mouth-to-mouth breathing and within a minute she regained consciousness, opened her eyes, and became aware of the people around her.

Why did my father's method work so easily? The reason is simple. When you drain the water out of the lungs by the force of gravity, you aerate the air sacs immediately and much more effectively—as long as it is done within the *reversible stages* of the "physiologic pathways of death." When you immediately begin giving mouth-to-mouth breathing to a drowning victim— as is the norm in our society—where is the large amount of water that is filling all of the air sacs in the lungs going to go? Unless the person's heart is still beating and the water can be immediately absorbed into the circulation, the chances of pulling that person through the 30-seconds-to-a-minute window of opportunity for survival are infinitely less with only mouth-to-mouth resuscitation. If the lungs are first drained, then and only then will the process of forced aeration, by blowing air into the lungs, be immediately effective and the "window of physiologic opportunity for survival" will not be lost.

When my brother Dariush stopped breathing and became catatonic from lack of oxygen, I am sure that relying only on mouth-to-mouth breathing would not have revived him. After 55 years, I still remember his rigid, cyanosed body. He probably had no more than 30 seconds left before he would have been irreversibly dead. Even if his body had survived, he would have suffered extensive brain damage.

At the time he drowned, no one knew about CPR. But, by Dariush being placed on the cook's back and having the cook run, the contents of Dariush's abdomen were pushed up and down against his diaphragm by the up and down movements of the cook's body. This, too, is a form of forced breathing, using the diaphragm, albeit at a more rapid rate. This method had an additional effect: by "gravity-draining" more blood into Dariush's heart, it too was stimulated into its normal rhythm and contractions.

I used CPR for the girl I treated because it was easier to do once her lungs were drained of all the water she had inhaled. This is a method I recommend to be used in future for drowned people who might still have a physiologic chance of living.

After 55 years, I still wonder how my father knew exactly what to do. He must have had unusually good common sense.

What You Need to Know About Choking

Both the esophagus and trachea (air pipe) begin at the back of the tongue, back to back. When we breathe, the air valve (epiglottis) at the back of the tongue and just above the voice box is open and air flows freely in and out. When we swallow, the tongue initiates the act by pushing the food or liquid that is about to be swallowed backwards in the direction of the opening of the esophagus. The backward push of the tongue prompts the epiglottis to close. In fact, the tongue in its backward contraction also pushes the "flap" of the valve down to make the "hole" watertight. Under normal circumstances, nothing can get down into the trachea when we swallow. We tend to take this marvel of design for granted. Now and then, some saliva, water, or a food particle might break the rule and enter the airway where it should not go! A spontaneous coughing reflex will blow the offending agent out of the bronchial tubes, from wherever it might have reached. This is the norm.

The unusual does sometimes occur, particularly if we begin to talk or breathe while chewing a mouthful of chunky food and confuse the reflex mechanisms between drawing in air to breathe or talk and swallowing the contents of the mouth. With the opening to the trachea wide open and the epiglottis not completely "flapped down," a food particle might find its way into the trachea. As we breathe in to initiate the cough reflex, we pull the particle further down. This is when the act of choking takes place.

Every year, a few thousand people choked to death as a result of this problem until a very intelligent medical doctor devised a way of using the already trapped air reserve in the lungs, putting it under a sudden pressure from outside, and forcing the obstructing particle out of the airways. The method is named after him and is called the Heimlich maneuver. Dr. Heimlich is world famous, and his method has saved tens of thousands of people since its introduction.

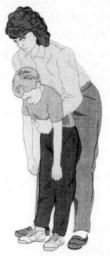

By a spontaneous tightening of the arms, the hands are drawn upward to force the contents of the abdomen against the diaphragm (Figure 14). In this way, the squeezed rib cage and diaphragm put the lungs and the air they contain under great pressure, enough to normally force the offending and misplaced particle to become a projectile. I am told the particle

Figure 14

exits the air passageway like a cork from a wine bottle. With young or old, the method is the same. You should practice this maneuver; you never know when it may be desperately needed.

Self-Treatment of Choking

What happens if you are alone and suddenly find yourself choking on a food particle and unable to breathe? What would you do? I asked myself this question and thought about it very carefully. I have devised a method that uses the same physical process. I have tried it many times to get practiced at it without the dangers of having a particle stuck in my throat. Let me introduce you to my "FB maneuver."

Firstly, one must realize that one has only about two minutes to save oneself. One must master the fact that to panic is counterproductive—one is bound to fail! Easier said than done when one's gag reflex is fully activated. But there is no other choice. The next step is to be alert enough to find a soft and bulky object like a small pillow or one's coat that can be rolled into a ball-like bundle. Next, kneel down on the ground. Then, roll up the pillow or bundle and hold it between your abdomen and your hands that grip each other at the wrists. The next step is the crucial one and one needs to practice it many times to develop an automatic reflex. With both hands gripping each other on the abdomen over the pillow, and while pressing the arms tightly into your side with elbows bent, *forcefully bend the upper part of the body against the thighs* (like the Islamic prayer position), thus forcing the hands and the pillow into the abdomen. This action puts enough pressure on the diaphragm and the chest wall to force the air out of the lungs with an extremely good chance of forcing the obstructing particle out of the bronchus or the trachea.

Practice the procedure gently, not forcefully, a few times at first so that you do not hurt yourself. You can harm yourself if you do the procedure on a full stomach or if you have heart problems. The best way to practice is to do it slowly and gently until you develop the knack. Breathe out but do not inhale when you bend down on your thighs. Let the air flow out freely. If you execute the procedure properly, you will feel the rush of air coming out of your mouth when you bend your body onto your thighs, with your hands and the pillow in between. *If you have the slightest suspicion that you may hurt yourself, do dry runs without forcing the pillow against your abdomen.*

8

Ideal Diet for Asthma, Allergies and Lupus

Chronic dehydration produces many symptoms, signs, and eventually, degenerative diseases. The physiological outcome of the sort of dehydration that produces any of the problems mentioned earlier in the book is almost the same. Different bodies manifest their early symptoms of drought differently, but in persistent dehydration that has been camouflaged by prescription medications, one by one the other symptoms and signs will kick in and eventually the person will suffer from multiple "diseases." You saw it in the case of Andrew Bauman. We in medicine have labeled these conditions as outright diseases or have grouped them as different "syndromes." In recent years, we have grouped some of the syndromes—with some typical blood tests—and called them autoimmune diseases, such as lupus, multiple sclerosis, muscular dystrophy, insulin-independent diabetes, and so on.

Medical research has until now been conducted on the assumption that many conditions—that I consider to be "states of dehydration or its complications"—are diseases of "unknown etiology." From the presently held perspectives of human health problems, one is not allowed to use the word "cure." You can at best "treat" a problem and hope it goes "into remission."

From my perspective, most painful degenerative diseases are states of local or regional drought—with varying patterns. It naturally follows that, once the drought is corrected, the problem will be cured if the dehydration damage is not extensive. I also believe that to evaluate "deficiency disorders"—water deficiency being one of them—one does not need to observe the same research protocols that are applied to the research of chemical products. Identifying the shortage and correcting the deficiency is all one has to do.

It is now clear that the treatment for all dehydration-produced conditions is the same—a single treatment protocol for umpteen number of conditions. Isn't that great? One program solves so many problems and avoids costly and unnecessary interferences with the body.

The first step in this treatment program involves a clear and determined upward adjustment of daily water intake. Persistent dehydration also causes a disproportionate loss of certain elements that should be adequately available in the stored reserves in the body. Naturally, the ideal treatment protocol will also involve an appropriate correction of the associated metabolic disturbance. In short, treatment of dehydration-produced diseases also involves correction of the secondary deficiencies that water deficiency imposes on some tissues of the body. This "multiple-deficiency" phenomenon, caused by dehydration, is at the root of many degenerative diseases, including lupus and cancer formation in the human body.

A change of lifestyle becomes vital for the correction of any dehydration-produced disorder. The backbone of the *water cure program* is, simply, sufficient water and salt intake; regular exercise; a balanced, mineral-rich diet that includes lots of fruits and vegetables, and the essential fats needed to make cell membranes, hormones, and nerve insulation; exclusion of caffeine and alcohol; meditation to solve and "detoxify" stressful thoughts; and exclusion of artificial sweeteners.

It should also be remembered that the sort of dehydration that manifests itself by the shortage of breath that is known to kill many thousands every year—asthma—leaves other "scars" within the interior parts of the human body. This is the reason asthma in childhood is a most devastating condition that will leave its mark on the child and will expose him or her to many different health problems in later life—such as in the case of Andrew Bauman, related earlier. My understanding of the serious damaging effects of dehydration during childhood is the reason I have been concentrating much of my efforts on the eradication of asthma among children.

The first nutrient the body needs is water. *Water is a nutrient*. It generates energy. Water dissolves all the minerals, proteins, starch, and other water-soluble components and, as blood, carries them around the body for distribution. Think of blood as sea water that has a few breeds of fish in it—red cells, white cells, platelets, proteins and enzymes that swim to a destination. The blood serum has almost the same mineral consistency and proportions as sea water.

The human body is in constant need of water. It is losing water through the lungs when we breathe out. It is losing water in perspiration, in urine production and in daily bowel movements. A good gauge for the water needs of the body is the color of urine. A well-hydrated person produces colorless urine—not counting the color of vitamins or color additives in food. A comparatively dehydrated person produces yellow urine. A truly dehydrated person produces urine that is orange in color.

The body needs no less than two quarts of water and some salt *every day* to compensate for its natural losses in urine, respiration and perspiration. (See Figure 15 on page 140.) Less than this amount will cause a burden on the kidneys. They will have to work harder to concentrate the urine and excrete as much chemical toxic wastes in as little water as possible. This process is most taxing to the kidneys, and this is why so many people end up needing dialysis in the final years of their drastically shortened lives. A rough rule of thumb for those who are heavyset is to drink a half ounce of water for every pound of body weight. A 200-lb person will need to take 100 ounces of water. Water should be taken anytime one is thirsty, even in the middle of a meal. Water intake in the middle of a meal does not drastically affect the process of digestion, but dehydration during food intake does. One should take at least two glasses of water first thing in the morning to correct for water loss during eight hours of sleep.

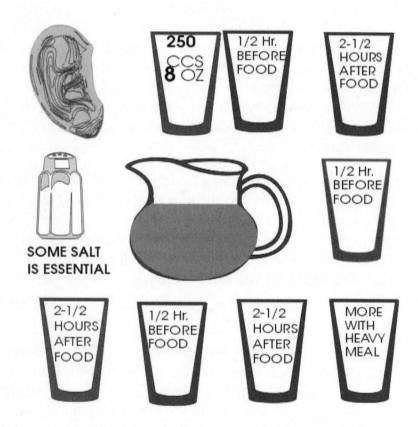

WATER SHOULD BE TAKEN **BEFORE FOOD**
TO PREVENT BLOOD CONCENTRATION

Figure 15

Minerals Are Vital

Certain minerals need to pass through the acidic environment of the stomach before they can be absorbed through the mucosa of the intestine. They are zinc, magnesium, manganese, selenium, iron, copper, chromium and molybdenum. The list is in the order, in my view, of each element's importance to the human body. The mineral elements that the body needs in largest quantities are sodium, potassium, calcium and magnesium. All one-a-day vitamin supplements are now composed in such a way that the daily requirements of the essential minerals—other than sodium, calcium and potassium—are provided in these tablets. The rest of the vital minerals are fully available in the variety of foods we eat. The reason why vitamin and mineral supplements are recommended is for "insurance" in case one's daily diet is not high quality and has an insufficient intake of fruits and vegetables.

The toxic mineral elements are mercury, lead, aluminum, arsenic, cadmium and, *in large quantities*, iron. These minerals should be avoided—they are absorbed better by the body if the stomach is less acidic than normal.

As we grow older, some of us manufacture less and less acid in our stomachs. The condition is called achlorhydria. People with achlorhydria can become deficient of vital minerals in their bodies. They also have difficulty in digesting meat.

In older cultures, eating pickles with food is a precautionary measure to prevent this problem. The use of vinegar in salads eaten with meals has the same effect, if the salad dressing is sour in taste. If the meal contains a lot of meat, the stomach normally secretes plenty of acid to break down the meat into small digestible particles that are then further reduced to the size of their amino acid components before they pass into the intestines and get absorbed. People who have difficulty digesting food should get into the habit of taking some lemon or pickles with their food.

Salt: The Eternal Medication

Salt is a vital substance for the survival of all living creatures, particularly humans, and especially people with asthma, allergies and autoimmune disease.

Salt is a "medication" used by healers throughout the ages. In certain cultures, salt is worth its weight in gold and is, in fact, exchanged weight for weight for gold. In desert countries, people know that salt intake is their insurance for survival. To these people, salt mines are synonymous with gold mines. Salt has a Biblical endorsement.

After many years of salt being bad-mouthed by ignorant health professionals and their media parrots, the importance of salt as a dietary supplement is once again being acknowledged and recognized. I was one of the early voices to bring about this change.

Water, salt and potassium together regulate the water content of the body. Water regulates the water content of the interior of the cell by working its way into all the cells it reaches. It has to get there to cleanse and extract the toxic waste of cell metabolism. Once water gets into the cells, the potassium content of the cells holds onto it and keeps it there—to the extent that potassium is available inside the cells. Even in the plant kingdom, it is potassium in the fruit that gives it firmness by holding water in the interior of the fruit. Our daily food contains ample potassium from its natural sources of fruits and vegetables, but not salt from its natural source. That is why we need to add salt to our daily diet.

Salt forces some water to keep it company outside the cells (osmotic retention of water by salt). It balances the amount of water that is held outside the cells.

Basically, there are two oceans of water in the body: one ocean is held <u>inside</u> the cells of the body and the other ocean is held <u>outside</u> the cells. Good health depends on a most delicate balance between the volume of these two oceans.

This balance is achieved by the regular intake of water, potassium-rich fruits and vegetables that also contain the vitamin needs of the body, and salt. Unrefined sea salt, which contains some of the other minerals that the body needs, is preferable.

When water is not available to get into the cells freely, it is filtered from the outside salty ocean and injected into the cells that are being overworked despite their water shortage. This secondary and emergency means of supplying important cells with "injected water" is the reason, in severe dehydration, that we develop edema and retain water. The design of our bodies is such that the extent of the ocean of water outside the cells is expanded to have the extra water available for filtration and emergency injection into vital cells. The brain commands an increase in salt and water retention by the kidneys. This directive of the brain is the reason we get edema when we don't drink enough water.

When water shortage in the body reaches a more critical level and "delivery of water" by its injection into the cells becomes the main route of supply to more and more cells, an associated rise in "injection pressure" becomes necessary. The significant rise in pressure needed to inject water into the cells becomes measurable and is labeled "hypertension."

Initially, the process of water filtration and its delivery into the cells is more efficient at night when the body is horizontal. The collected water, which settles mostly in the legs during the day, does not have to fight the force of gravity to get into the blood circulation when the body is horizontal. If reliance on this process of emergency hydration of some cells continues for long, the lungs begin to get waterlogged at night and breathing becomes difficult. The person needs more pillows to sit upright to sleep. This condition is called "cardiac asthma" and it is the consequence of dehydration. However, in this condition you must not overload the system by drinking too much water at the beginning. Increases in water intake must be slow and spaced out—until urine production begins to increase at the same rate that you drink water.

When we drink enough water to pass clear urine, we also pass out a lot of the salt that was held back. This is how we can get rid of edema fluid from the body: by drinking more water. Not diuretics, but more water! Water is the best natural diuretic that exists.

In a person who has extensive edema and whose heart sometimes has irregular or very rapid beats with little effort, the increase in water intake should be gradual and spaced out, but water should not be withheld from the body. Salt intake should be limited for two or three days because the *body is still in an overdrive mode to retain it*. Once the edema has cleared up, salt should *not* be withheld from the body.

Salt: Some of Its Hidden Miracles

Salt has many other functions than just regulating the water content of the body. Here are some of its additional important functions in the body:

- Salt is a strong natural antihistamine. It can be used to relieve asthma by putting it on the tongue after drinking a glass or two of water. It is as effective as an inhaler, without the toxicity. You should drink one or two glasses of water before putting salt on the tongue.

- Salt is a strong "anti-stress" element for the body.

- Salt is vital for extracting excess acidity from inside the cells, particularly the brain cells. If you don't want Alzheimer's disease, don't go salt-free, and don't let *them* put you on diuretic medications for long!

- Salt is vital for the kidneys to clear excess acidity and pass the acidity into the urine. Without sufficient salt in the body, the body will become more and more acidic.

- Salt is essential in the treatment of emotional and affective disorders. Lithium is a salt substitute that is used in the treatment of depression. To prevent suffering from depression, make sure you take some salt.

- Salt is essential for preserving the serotonin and melatonin levels in the brain. When water and salt perform their natural antioxidant duties and clear the toxic waste from the body, essential amino acids, such as tryptophan and tyrosine, will not be sacrificed as chemical antioxidants. In a well-hydrated body, tryptophan is spared and gets into the brain tissue where it is used to manufacture serotonin, melatonin, and tryptamine—essential antidepression neurotransmitters.

- Salt, in my opinion, is vital for the *prevention and treatment of cancer.* Cancer cells are killed by oxygen; they are anaerobic "organisms." They must live in a low-oxygen environment. When the body is well hydrated and salt expands the volume of blood circulation to reach all parts of the body, the oxygen and the active and "motivated" immune cells in the blood reach the cancerous tissue and destroy it. As I explained in the section on lupus, dehydration—shortage of water and salt—suppresses the immune system and its disease-fighting cells' activity in the body.

- Salt is vital for maintaining muscle tone and strength. Lack of bladder control in those who suffer from involuntary leakage of urine could be a consequence of low salt intake. The following letter from Dottlee Reid, in her sixties, speaks volumes. It shows how salt intake helped her get over her constant problem of involuntary leakage of urine. I have chosen to print this letter here to share with millions of senior citizens in America the good news that adequate *salt* intake can possibly save them from the embarrassment of having to constantly wear pads. She has given me permission to print her address and telephone number for those who wish to verify her story.

2203 Camelia Circle
Baytown, TX 77520
Nov. 27, 1999

Dear Doctor Batmanghelidj:

"June 25, 1999 I had to go home from work because the pain in my knee became unbearable. (This was an old wound years ago caused by a chiropractor that had been bruised again.) I was staying in bed a lot as it was too painful to try to walk.

Thank God Global Health Solutions got my name and address from somewhere and I got your book (Your Body's Many Cries For Water) and tapes. By July 3, 1999 I decided to try and walk around the block. I made it and July 4, 1999 I walked six blocks to church. On July 5, 1999 I rode seven hours only stopping twice to use the rest room. I have a very weak bladder and had even taken spare clothing as I was sure they would be needed. I arrived with not a drop of anything on my clothing, and for the first time in my life I was not tired and I even took a walk before I went to bed.

I was very thin and was limited on what I could eat. Suddenly I find I am eating things I have not been able to eat in years— peaches, canteloupe, watermelon, tomatoes, pineapple and even sweets—and I was enjoying them with no side effects.

I had not been drinking anything, but water for years, but I had talked myself off salt. A bad mistake! My muscles were really screaming as well as many parts of my body.

I still have problems to be worked out, but I'm learning how to listen to my own body and I hope to see the day I won't have anymore problems with gas, digestion, circulation and allergies.

I can truthfully say most days I do feel better than I have in man
years and I can never thank you enough for your help.

May God bless you as you try to help those He has placed on
this earth.

> *Gratefully Yours*
> *Dottlee Reid*
> *Phone 281-422-4522*

☞ ☞ ☞ ☞ ☞

- Salt is most effective in stabilizing irregular heartbeats and, contrary to the misconception that it causes high blood pressure, it is actually essential for the regulation of blood pressure—in conjunction with water. ***Naturally, the proportions are critical.*** A low-salt diet with high water intake will, in some people, actually cause the blood pressure to rise. ***As a secondary complication, it can also cause asthma-like shortness of breath***. The logic is simple. If you drink water and do not take salt, the water will not stay in the blood circulation adequately to completely fill all the blood vessels. In some, this will cause fainting, and in some, it will cause tightening of the arteries—***and eventually constriction of bronchioles in the lungs***—to the point of registering a rise in blood pressure, complicated by breathlessness. One or two glasses of water and some salt— a little of it on the tongue—will quickly and efficiently quieten a racing and "thumping" heart, ***and in the long run***, will reduce the blood pressure and cure breathlessness.

- Salt is vital for sleep regulation. It is a natural hypnotic. If you drink a full glass of water, then put a few grains of salt on your tongue, and let it stay there, you will fall into a natural, deep sleep. Don't use salt on your tongue unless you also drink water. Repeated use of salt by itself might cause nose bleeds.

- Salt is a vitally needed element in the treatment of

diabetics. It helps balance the sugar levels in the blood and reduces the need for insulin in those who have to inject the chemical to regulate their blood sugar levels. Water and salt reduce the extent of secondary damage associated with diabetes.

- Salt is vital for the generation of hydroelectric energy in all of the cells in the body. It is used for local power generation at the sites of energy need by the cells.

- Salt is vital to the communication and information processing of nerve cells the entire time that the brain cells work—from the moment of conception to death.

- Salt is vital for the absorption of food particles through the intestinal tract.

- Salt is vital for clearing the lungs of mucus plugs and sticky phlegm, particularly in asthma, emphysema and cystic fibrosis sufferers.

- Salt on the tongue will stop persistent dry coughs.

- Salt is vital for clearing up catarrh and sinus congestion.

- Salt is vital for the prevention of gout and gouty arthritis.

- Salt is essential for the prevention of muscle cramps.

- Salt is vital in preventing excess saliva production to the point that it flows out of the mouth during sleep. Needing to constantly mop up excess saliva indicates salt shortage.

- Osteoporosis, in a major way, is the result of salt and water shortage in the body.

- Salt is absolutely vital to making the structure of bones firm.

- Salt is vital for maintaining self-confidence and a positive self-image—a serotonin- and melatonin-controlled "personality output."

- Salt is vital for maintaining sexuality and libido.

- Salt is vital for reducing a double chin. When the body is short of salt, it means the body really is short of water. The salivary glands sense the salt shortage and are obliged to produce more saliva to lubricate the act of chewing and swallowing and also to supply the stomach with water that it needs for breaking down foods. Circulation to the salivary glands increases and the blood vessels become "leaky" in order to supply the glands with more water to manufacture saliva. This "leakiness" spills to areas beyond the glands themselves, causing increased bulk under the skin of the chin, the cheeks, and into the neck.

- Salt is vital for preventing varicose veins and spider veins on the legs and thighs.

- Sea salt contains about 80 mineral elements that the body needs. Some of these elements are needed in trace amounts. Unrefined sea salt is a better choice of salt than other types of salt on the market. Ordinary table salt that is bought in the supermarkets has been stripped of its companion elements and contains additive elements such as aluminum silicate to keep it powdery and porous. Aluminum is a very toxic element in our nervous system. It is implicated as one of the primary causes of Alzheimer's disease.

- As much as salt is good for the body in asthma, excess potassium is bad for it. Too much orange juice, too many bananas, or any "sports drink" containing too much potassium might precipitate an asthma attack, particularly if too much of the drink or too many bananas are taken before exercising. It can cause an exercise-induced asthma attack. To prevent such attacks, some salt intake before exercise will increase the lungs' capacity for air exchange. It will also decrease excess sweating.

It is a good policy to add some salt to orange juice to balance the actions of sodium and potassium in maintaining the required

.olume of water inside and outside the cells. In some cultures, salt is added to melon and other fruits to accentuate their sweetness. In effect, these fruits contain mostly potassium. By adding salt to them before eating, a balance between the intake of sodium and potassium results. The same should be done to other juices.

I received a call one day from one of the readers of my book to tell me how he had unwittingly hurt his son. Knowing that orange juice was full of vitamin C, he forced his son to drink several glasses of it every day. In the meantime, the young boy developed breathing problems and had a number of asthma attacks until he reached college and moved out of the sphere of influence of his father. His asthma cleared and his breathing became normal. The father told me he had to call his son and apologize for having given him such a hard time when he was younger. The more the son had rebelled against orange juice, the more the father had insisted he should take it, convinced a large amount was good for him.

As a rough rule of thumb, you need about 3 grams of salt—a half-teaspoon—for every 10 glasses of water, or a quarter teaspoon per quart of water You should take salt throughout the day. If you exercise and sweat, you need more salt. In hot climates, you need to take even more salt. In these climates, salt makes the difference between survival and better health and heat exhaustion and death.

Warning! **You must at the same time not overdo salt.** You must observe the ratio of salt and water needs of the body. You must always make sure you drink enough water to wash the excess salt out of the body. *If your weight suddenly goes up in one day, you have taken too much salt.* Hold back on salt intake for one day and drink plenty of water to increase your urine output and get rid of your swelling.

Those in heart failure—or kidney failure needing dialysis—MUST consult with their doctors before increasing their salt intake.

If you begin to drink water according to my protocol, you might also benefit from taking a one-a-day vitamin tablet daily, particularly if you do not exercise or eat hearty portions of vegetables and fruits. Meat and fish proteins are good sources of selenium and zinc. If you are under stress, and until it is over, you might consider adding some vitamin B6 and zinc to your diet in addition to what is available in the vitamin tablets.

If you suffer from cold-sores (herpes simplex virus on the lips and even in the eyes) or genital herpes, make sure you add zinc and vitamin B6 to your diet. <u>Your viral sores might very well be the result of zinc deficiency and its associated complications</u>.

Proteins

Experts are of the opinion that the body needs a minimum of between 1.1 and 1.4 grams of good-quality protein for every kilogram—2.2 pounds—of body weight per day. A 200-lb (90 kg) person needs about 4.5 ounces—120 grams—of protein a day to maintain his or her muscle mass. At this level of protein intake, the body will retain its normal composition of protein reserves and will not break into them and deplete some of the amino acid reserves.

Children need a basic minimum of about 1 gram of protein for every pound of body weight.

In advanced societies that have high demands on their labor force for increased productivity, and have no food shortages, the recommended regular intake of protein seems to be around 10 ounces per day. The more physically active you are, the more protein-containing food your body needs. The extra protein is needed for tissue repairs and the manufacture of enzymes and neurotransmitters. High-protein diets are now fashionable in weight-loss programs.

Good-quality proteins can be found in eggs, milk, and legumes, such as lentils that are 24 percent high-quality protein, mung beans, broad beans, soya beans and tofu (extract of soya bean). Vegetables also contain good-quality protein (spinach is about 13 percent protein), as do fresh turkey, chicken, veal, beef, pork and fish. I use the word "fresh" because animal meat contains different enzymes that quickly destroy some of the essential amino acids within its proteins. Prolonged exposure to oxygen also destroys some of the essential amino acids in meat proteins. It makes the good fats in meat rancid and useless to the body. This is why in old cultures such as Chinese, Jewish, and Muslim, meat and fish have to be from a freshly killed source.

Do not take individual amino acids as supplements. At a certain concentration, some have adverse effects on the mineral and vitamin balance of the body. Amino acids in the body function more efficiently when they are "proportionately" represented.

Eggs

Eggs are a wholesome food. An average egg weighs 50 grams and has an energy value of 80 calories. The white of an egg weighs about 33 grams and the yolk about 17 grams. Eggs contain about 6 grams of top-quality proteins, no carbohydrates and no fiber. The protein content of eggs is composed of a balanced range of amino acids. Eggs are rich in vitamins such as biotin, and minerals such as manganese, selenium, phosphorus and copper. The yolk is a rich source of sulphur, a natural antioxidant that is now recognized as being vital for health and well-being.

About 10 percent of an egg is its lipid or fat content. The lipid composition of the egg yolk is unique. It is rich in both lecithin, which is the precursor of the neurotransmitter acetylcholine, and DHA (docosa-hexa-enoic acid). DHA is a most essential fat for maintaining brain function. It is needed for the constant repair of brain cell membranes and their cell-to-cell contact points— synaptosomes. The nerve structure of the eyes uses much DHA for interpreting colors and for quality and sharpness of vision.

Apart from being found in eggs, DHA is also found in cold-water fish and algae.

It is being increasingly understood that the level of cholesterol in the circulation is not affected by a high egg diet. It is a medically published fact that an elderly man has for many years eaten about 24 eggs a day without any clinically significant rise in his cholesterol level.

There is no such thing as bad cholesterol! There are only uninformed and ignorant ideas that are exploited commercially.

The next time you come across a person who talks about "bad cholesterol" being the cause of heart disease, ask him or her: "Is it not true that we measure the cholesterol levels in the body from blood that is drawn from a vein?" If it is true that the level of cholesterol is the cause of plaques and obstruction of the blood vessels, when a slower rate of blood flow would encourage further cholesterol deposits, then we should also get more blockage of veins of the body. Since there is not a single scientific report of cholesterol deposits causing blockage of the veins, the assumption that cholesterol is "bad" and is the cause of heart disease is erroneous and unscientific. It is a commercial hype to sell drugs and medical services.

Let me explain why we get cholesterol deposits in the arteries of the heart or the brain or even on the inner wall of the major arteries of the body. Remember, when we say "dehydration" it really means concentrated, acidic blood. Acidic blood that is also concentrated pulls water out of the cells lining the arterial wall. At the same time, the fast rush of blood against the delicate cells lining the inner wall of the arteries, weakened by loss of their water and damaged by constant toxicity of concentrated blood, produces microscopic abrasions.

Another of the many functions of cholesterol is its use as a "waterproof dressing" to cover the damaged sites within the arterial membranes until they are repaired. Cholesterol acts as a "grease gauze" that protects the wall of the artery from rupturing and peeling off. When you look at cholesterol through this perspective, you will realize what a blessing it really is.

In my opinion, all the statistics about the level of cholesterol in the blood and the number of people who die of heart disease reflect the extent of the killer dehydration that has also caused the level of blood cholesterol to rise.

I will discuss another most important role of cholesterol in the body later in this chapter. Based on my researched understanding of cholesterol, I have no hesitation in recommending eggs as a very good source of the essential dietary needs of the human body.

Milk Products

For people who can digest milk, natural, unsweetened yogurt is a good source of high-quality protein. It also contains lots of vitamins and good bacteria. The good bacteria in yogurt keep the intestinal tract healthy and help prevent the growth of toxic bacteria and toxic yeasts such as candida. Of course, people who are allergic to dairy products should not take yogurt.

Cheeses are also a good source of protein. Freshly prepared cheeses are easier to digest and, in my opinion, are more wholesome than aged cheeses.

Some people cannot digest cow's milk easily. Soya milk is a very good substitute. If you do not like the taste of soya milk, mix it with carrot juice and enjoy the advantage of additional vitamins and nutrients. The combination is healthy and tasty.

Fats

Fat is an essential dietary requirement of the body. Some vital fatty acids that make up certain fats and oils are used as primary materials in the manufacture of cell membranes. They are also primary ingredients from which many of the hormones of the body are manufactured. The manufacture of sex hormones depends on the presence of some essential fats in the body, including the much maligned cholesterol. Nerve cells need the "good" fats to remanufacture the constantly-used-up nerve endings.

The essential fat components are omega 6—a polyunsaturated fatty acid known as Linoleic acid—and omega 3—a super unsaturated fatty acid known as alpha-Linolenic acid. These fatty acids are in the form of oils. Our bodies cannot make these essential fatty acids and have to import them in the form of oils in food.

The average body needs, <u>absolutely</u>, between 6 and 9 grams of Linoleic acid (omega 6) a day. It also needs around 2 to 9 grams of alpha-Linolenic acid (omega 3), the most essential of the fatty acids. These fatty acids are needed particularly by the brain cells and their long nerves to manufacture insulated membranes that need to be impermeable and prevent interference to the rate and flow of neurotransmission. The nerve endings in the retina that are involved in object recognition and clarity of sight have a high turnover of these essential fatty acids, particularly DHA. DHA is made from omega 3 fatty acid and is vital for brain cell composition. People with neurological disorders have been shown to be short of DHA.

As mentioned, eggs, cold-water fish and algae are good sources of DHA. Another excellent source of the omega 3 and omega 6 fatty acids, in an ideal ratio of 3 to 1, is flaxseed (also know as linseed) oil that is cold-pressed and bottled in dark containers that keep out light. Light destroys these essential oils, which is why they are also packed in dark capsules. Sesame oil has the desirable property of being highly unsaturated. It is the eating oil of choice in many ancient cultures. Canola oil is also a good source of some essential fatty acids. The reason oils are better than solid fats is because at normal body temperature they remain as oils and do not turn into sticky lard.

For detailed information on the essential fatty acids and their best sources, refer to the book, *Fats that Heal, Fats that Kill,* by Dr. Udo Erasmus. The book's ISBN is 0-920470-38-6. If you are health conscious, you need to read this book. Another good and readable book on this topic is *Smart Fats,* by Dr. Michael A. Schmidt (ISBN 1-883319-62-5).

Butter is a rich source of fat-soluble vitamins, such as vitamin K, vitamin A, vitamin E, lecithin, folic acid, and more. Butter is also a rich source of calcium and phosphorous. The body needs some fat in its daily diet. You cannot go fat-free and survive for long. The body is not able to manufacture certain fat components that are needed to make its insulating membranes. If you don't give the body what it needs, it will try to make the required element from the carbohydrate content in its daily diet. However, since the body is unable to complete the process of making "essential fats," it proceeds to store the unfinished product. This is how some people grow disproportionately fat. If you want to lose weight, your diet must contain some fat. Each gram of fat provides the body with 9 calories of energy.

Fruits, Vegetables and Sunlight

The body also needs fruits and green vegetables daily. They are ideal sources of the natural vitamins and essential minerals we need. Green vegetables also contain a great deal of beta-carotenes and even some DHA fatty acid needed by the brain. Fruits and vegetables are important for maintaining the pH balance of the body. Chlorophyll contains a very high quantity of magnesium. Magnesium is to chlorophyll what iron is to hemoglobin in the blood—an oxygen carrier. In the human body, magnesium is the bonding anchor to the energy-storing unit within the cell membranes all over the body. The unit is called magnesium-adenosine-triphosphate (MgATP). If water reaches the MgATP pool and is enzymatically positioned to break it down, lots of energy will be released—the formula is presented in the section on lupus.

To asthmatics, sunlight is "medicine." Light from the sun acts on the cholesterol deposits on the skin and converts them to Vitamin D. Vitamin D encourages bone making and the entrapment of calcium by the bones—which in children helps them grow. Vitamin D also stimulates calcium absorption in the intestinal tract. Calcium has a direct acid-neutralizing effect in the body and is effective in balancing the cell pH—an outcome that helps alleviate asthma complications.

If you drink adequate amounts of water every day, take the required amount of salt, and get plenty of exercise—preferably in the open air and under good light—your body will begin to adjust its own intake of proteins and carbohydrates, as well as its fat requirements to use for energy. Your need for proteins will increase. Your need for carbohydrates will decrease and your fat-burning enzymes will consume more fat than is in the average diet. Contrary to the belief that cholesterol cannot be metabolized once it is deposited, that too will be cleared. The cholesterol deposits in the arteries may take longer to disappear than you might wish, but the body has all the chemical know-how to clear cholesterol plaques.

I repeat, there is no such thing as "bad" cholesterol. Remember that cholesterol is vital to body physiology. We have to find out why the body manufactures more of it than usual. The following explanation is one of many I have found for this.

When there is a shortage of water in the body, less hydroelectric energy is manufactured to energize *all* the dependent functions—like the low water flow in the river that feeds an electricity-generating dam. After a while, the dam will not hold enough water to operate all the generators. In real-life situations, when cheap energy from hydroelectric dams is insufficient, power generators begin to burn oil or coal to generate electricity.

In the body, the alternative source of energy is from calcium deposits in the bone or inside the cells. The energy trapped in the union of two calcium molecules that are fused together is used instead. For each two calcium molecules bonded together, one unit of ATP energy is also trapped. The cells in the body have much trapped calcium in different storage sites that become broken up and their energy is used. There comes a time when this process results in an availability of too many loose calcium molecules—fuel ash. Fortunately, "calcium ash" is easily recycled.

As I already mentioned, sunlight—energy—converts cholesterol in the skin to vitamin D. Vitamin D is responsible for facilitating the re-entrapment of calcium and its reentry into the cells to be rebonded. Vitamin D sticks to its receptors on the cell membrane and, simultaneously, one unit of calcium attaches itself to the exposed tail of the vitamin D in the process of entering the cell through the cell membrane. The union of calcium with vitamin D to the membrane receptor acts as a "magnetic rod" and a whole chain of other essential elements and amino acids stick to the exposed calcium and are drawn into the cell.

In this way, the energy of sunlight and its conversion of cholesterol to vitamin D has a direct physiological impact on the feeding of the cells of the body. When calcium reenters the cell, it takes other essential elements with it into the cell. In this way, the cell receives raw materials for repair and energy metabolism. At the same time, the surplus energy that enters the cell is used to fuse together calcium molecules and once again store energy in the calcium "bondage" for future use.

Once you understand the logic behind the "cascade" of the chemical events in the body, you will realize the vital importance of cholesterol to cell metabolism and the health of the cell.

You should put the higher cholesterol levels of the body to full use. Make more vitamin D from it and promote better-functioning and fully utilized cells in your body. Use sunlight to your advantage to lower your cholesterol. Some of you might immediately react negatively to this statement and express your fear of melanoma. It is my belief that cancers in the body are produced by dehydration, inactivity, bad choice of foods and wrong beverages. For over 20 years, I played three hours of tennis, six days a week, in the heat of the early afternoon sun in Tehran. I did not develop any form of cancer.

You cannot sit at a desk in an artificially lit office and expect to have a normal cholesterol level in your body. And in this situation, you will probably have a health professional, who does not understand the mechanisms and relationships of sunlight energy conversion, label this natural outcome of an incomplete chain of metabolic events as a "disease," and a vital element, cholesterol, will be labeled as "bad."

Exercise

The most important factor for survival, after air, water, salt and food, is exercise. Exercise is more important to the health of the individual than sex, entertainment or anything else that might be pleasurable. The following points explain the importance of exercise for better health and pain-free longer life.

- Exercise expands the vascular system in the muscle tissue and prevents hypertension.

- It opens the capillaries in the muscle tissue and, by lowering the resistance to blood flow in the arterial system, causes the blood pressure to drop to normal.

- Exercise builds up muscle mass and prevents the muscles being broken down as fuel.

- Exercise stimulates the activity of fat-burning enzymes for manufacture of the constantly needed energy for muscle activity. When you train, you are in effect changing the source of energy for muscle activity. You convert the energy source from sugar that is in circulation to fat that is stored in the muscle itself.

- Exercise makes muscles burn as additional fuel some of the amino acids that would otherwise reach toxic levels in the body. In their more-than-normal levels in the blood— usually reached in an unexercised body—certain branched-chain amino acids cause a drastic destruction and depletion of other vital amino acids. Some of these discarded essential amino acids are constantly needed by the brain to manufacture its neurotransmitters. Two of these essential amino acids are tryptophan and tyrosine. The brain uses trytophan to make serotonin, melatonin, tryptamine and indoleamine, all of which are antidepressants and regulate sugar level and blood pressure. Tyrosine is used for the manufacture of adrenaline, noradrenaline and dopamine—vital for the coordination of body physiology when it has to take a physical action, such as fighting, running, playing sports, and so on. Excess tyrosine loss from the amino acid reserves of the body is also a primary factor in Parkinson's disease.

- Unexercised muscle gets broken down. As a result of the excretion of muscle parts from the body, some of the reserves of zinc and vitamin B6 also get lost. At a certain stage of this constant depletion of vitamin B6 and zinc, certain mental disorders and neurological complications occur. In effect, this happens in autoimmune diseases, including lupus and muscular dystrophy.

- Exercise makes the muscles hold more water in reserve and prevent increased concentration of blood that would otherwise damage the lining of the blood vessel walls.

- Exercise lowers blood sugar in diabetics and decreases their need for insulin or tablet medications.

- Exercise compels the liver to manufacture sugar from the fat that it stores or the fat that is circulating within the blood.

- Exercise causes an increase in the mobility of the joints in the body. It causes the creation of an intermittent vacuum inside the joint cavities. The force of the vacuum causes suction of water into the cavity. Water in the joint cavity brings dissolved nutrients to the cells inside the cartilage. Increased water content of the cartilage also adds to its lubrication and smoother bone-on-bone gliding movements of the joint.

• Leg muscles act as secondary hearts. By their contractions and relaxations during the time we are upright, the leg muscles overcome the force of gravity. They pump into the venous system the blood that was sent to the legs. Because of the pressure breakers—and one-directional valves in the vein—the blood in the leg veins is pushed upward against gravity by frequent contraction of the leg muscles. This is how the leg muscles act as hearts for the venous system in the body. This is a value to exercise that not many people appreciate. Leg muscles also cause an equally effective flow within the lymphatic system and cause edema in the legs to disappear.

• Exercise strengthens the bones of the body and helps prevent osteoporosis.

• Exercise increases the production of all vital hormones, enhancing libido and heightening sexual performance.

• One hour of walking will cause the activation of fat-burning enzymes, which remain active for 12 hours. A morning and afternoon walk will keep these enzymes active round the clock and will cause clearance of cholesterol deposits in the arterial system.

• Exercise will enhance the activity of the adrenaline-operated sympathetic nerve system. Adrenaline will also reduce the oversecretion of histamine and, as a result, will prevent asthma attacks and allergic reactions—providing the body is fully hydrated.

- Exercise will increase production of endorphins and enkephalins, the natural opiates of the body. They produce the same "high" that drug addicts try to achieve through their abusive intake.

What Are the Best Forms of Exercise?

Exercising the body for endurance is better than exercising it for speed or for building excess muscle. In selecting an exercise, you should consider its lifetime value. A long-distance runner will enjoy the exercise value of long-distance runs into old age. A sprinter will not sprint for exercise at a later phase of life.

The best exercise that one can benefit from even to a ripe old age, and without causing damage to the joints, is walking. Other exercises that will increase one's endurance are swimming, golf, skiing, skating, climbing, tennis, squash, bicycling, tai chi, dancing and aerobics. In selecting an exercise, one should evaluate its ability to keep the fat-burning enzymes active for longer durations. Outdoor forms of exercise are more beneficial for the body than indoor forms of exercise. The body becomes better connected to "nature."

The four most vital steps to better health (Figure 16)—balancing the water and salt content of the body, exercising the muscle mass of the body, taking a balanced daily diet of proteins and vegetables, and avoiding dehydrating beverages—are shown on the following page.

FOUR NATURAL STEPS

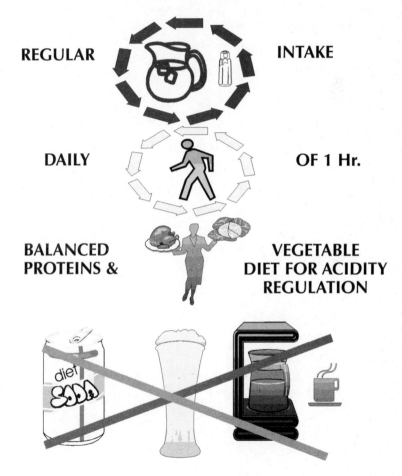

REGULAR INTAKE

DAILY OF 1 Hr.

BALANCED PROTEINS & VEGETABLE DIET FOR ACIDITY REGULATION

Figure 16

"You cannot by reasoning correct
a man of ill opinion which by
reasoning he never acquired."
                              Francis Bacon

9

Quality of Drinking Water

Naturally, the quality of drinking water is most important to health. Water should be water and not just any drink. Asthmatics should observe this instruction to the letter. Water should be free of chemicals, particularly caffeine and alcohol.

Please bear in mind that caffeine and alcohol are toxic chemicals—addictive drugs—as far as the cells of the human body are concerned. It is true that the manufacturers of these agents have unrestricted permission to contaminate good drinking water with these toxic chemicals and to sell them to the public, but, sooner or later, their detrimental impact on society will also become the focus of attention like the tobacco industry presently is.

It is my sincere belief that many of our society's problems of ill health can be blamed on the marketing tactics and unceasing push of the beverage industry. They tend to cultivate the palates of younger people toward the selection and use of their products in preference to the water that young bodies need to develop naturally and normally. Once teenagers—the target of the industry—become addicted to caffeine, the industry has converted them to cash machines for the rest of their shortened lives! The unfortunate outcome of addiction to caffeine is the "upgrade" effect that forces some children to experiment with harder drugs.

Caffeine is a natural diuretic. It forces more water out of the body than is contained in the caffeinated beverage. Caffeine also acts directly on the brain cells and forces them to use some of their critical energy reserves on trivial actions and whims. It lowers the threshold for triggering an action from cells that would otherwise remain quiet until a more serious engagement is deemed necessary. The effect of caffeine on the brain is energy depletion. Caffeine, if taken repeatedly, eventually exhausts the brain. When the brain needs energy reserves to cope with a crisis, it will be far less effective because it is energy-depleted and depressed. The energy-reserve-depleting effect of caffeine on the brain is one of the primary causes of Attention Deficit Disorder (ADD).

Caffeine has another detrimental effect on the brain that should be considered as the second main impact that pushes the brain in the direction of reaching an ADD status. The brain maintains its energy reserves to use for new confrontations, experiences, dangers, and exciting, fresh ideas. This is how it learns selectively and from new experiences. Caffeine not only depletes the stored energy pools in the brain, it also inhibits the enzyme system initiated by PD (phospho-diesterase). PD activity is a vital step in "memory making" by the brain cells.

All seeds that are designed to create the next generation of a plant contain in their covering shell one or other chemical to deter food scavengers, such as ants and beetles, from eating the protein-rich seeds before they sprout. If this were not so, these plants would become extinct. Legumes such as lentils, peas and green beans possess a chemical called CCK (chol-e-cysto-kinin), a digestive enzyme inhibitor that causes a form of indigestion in the systems of critters that eat the seeds. It causes gas formation in humans who eat lentils without soaking them well and discarding the skin, or boiling them briefly first, washing them well, and then boiling them a second time until cooked. This is the way to "de-gas" legumes that would normally produce indigestion. Get rid of the CCK.

Caffeine is *naturally designed to cause stupefaction of the brain*. Caffeine is used by a number of plants as a nerve warfare chemical against their predators. The coffee plant produces caffeine in its seeds to defend itself. Caffeine inhibits the nervous system and the memory mechanisms in its "food-chain" predators in such a way that they lose their "wit" and their art of camouflage. They become less alert and less reactive, and thus less able to protect themselves. They become much easier prey for their own predators.

That is why the coffee plant is plagued by far fewer bugs than most other plants during its growth period. Bugs know better than to eat it. But we humans take the caffeine-containing coffee beans, brew them to our desired concentration, and consume the plant's chemical poison as a pleasure-inducing beverage. High soda consumption, in my opinion, is the reason so many kids in American schools have reading and learning problems. Despite all the money that is spent on their education, their average standard is far below children in less-privileged societies, whose access to caffeine-containing beverages is much more limited.

The beverage industry grows and thrives on the addictive properties of caffeine. A report published in the magazine, *The Nation*, April 27, 1998, states: "The most conservative estimates have children and teens guzzling more than sixty-four gallons of soda a year—an amount that has tripled for teens since 1978, doubled for the 6-11 set and increased by a quarter for under-5 tots (from a 1994 survey by the Agriculture Department)." This finding confirms what I published several years ago in my book, *Your Body's Many Cries for Water,* on pages 104–113. It is also interesting to note that the increased consumption of sodas by infants under five years is most probably why the rate of asthma occurrence in that age group tripled in the years between 1980 and 1994.

The beverage industry's recent name selection of new brands—Surge, Zapped, Full Speed, Outburst, Josta, laced with caffeine and the pick-me-up herb, guarana, that hypes "raw primal power"—is designed to attract children and teenagers to consume more and more sodas. The 12-oz cans of soda that contain high amounts of caffeine include Jolt with 72 mg., XTC with 70 mg., Pepsi-Cola's Josta with 58 mg., and Coca-Cola's Surge with 51 mg. And you get a near double dose when you buy the 20-oz bottles.

At schools, the kids often take sodas in place of milk and the schools profit from the sale of these addictive beverages. They serve the regular 12-oz cans of soda, with Mountain Dew containing 55 mg. of caffeine per can, Coke containing 45 mg., Sunkist with 40 mg., and Pepsi with 37 mg.

Grown-ups consume so much coffee that coffee bars are growing like mushrooms. It is said that a 12-oz cup of regular Starbucks coffee contains 190 mg. of caffeine.

It is my professional opinion that caffeine by itself has all the detrimental effects on the brain cells to produce the type of brain physiology that dislocates the brain from stimuli received from outside. In addition, the dehydration caused by extensive caffeine intake produces different health problems, devastatingly and early. Among the symptoms are asthma and allergies. Thus, my protocol for the treatment of asthma excludes any form of caffeine-containing beverage until the body has recovered from caffeine's unhealthy side effects, particularly on the brain and its nervous system. After that, wisdom will have to take over.

Artificial Sweetener Disease

One of the falsehoods that society has to correct is the assumption that the human brain can be tricked into doing things that are against its inner intelligence. Something that has had a devastating impact on our society is the introduction of artificial sweeteners to enhance the taste of food and drink without the energy content of the natural sugars that the palate is accustomed to. We do not realize that the brain is a very sensitive "computer" that tabulates the energy content of any "sweetness" in its command and control functions. We think we can fool it by giving it sweetness without the customary food values associated with something sweet. If these are your thoughts, you are only fooling yourself, not your brain! You misinform your conscious mind and cause it to split from the natural inner design and wisdom installed in your brain.

Blood sugar levels are constantly monitored and adjusted according to the rules of supply and demand established in each body. When you stimulate the taste buds with sweetness, the brain assumes that real sugar is being consumed and it calculates the quantity of energy that has entered the body. If the amount of "sugar" that has entered the system is going to upset the preset levels, the liver is instructed to switch from a sugar-manufacturing mode to a sugar-storing mode. Here the roller-coaster effects of false sweetness on the body physiology begin. The liver begins to mop up the roaming sugar from the blood circulation, "thinking" that more will enter it from the gut. Since the "promised" sugar needed to keep the blood sugar levels within the norm is not forthcoming, the actual blood sugar levels will start to drop. This is when the panic begins—even before a marked drop in the levels of the blood sugar has occurred.

The brain chemistry of someone in a state of "sweetener panic" will compel that person to seek food and eat more than normal, even a short time after a meal! Some people who are determined to lose weight might fight the urge to eat and might reach for another soda—exactly what the beverage industry wants people to do. Hence the rise in the sale of sodas and the increase in the number of people who are fat! No fewer than 30 percent of the American people are grossly overweight.

The artificial sweetener, aspartame, used in over 5,000 food products is considered to have many adverse effects in the human body, other than the weight problem I have mentioned. Dr. H. J. Roberts, F.A.C.P., F.C.C.P., has identified a number of health problems caused by aspartame and calls them "aspartame disease." He thinks that all the problems attributed to silicone breast implants that caused the bankruptcy of Dow Corning were in fact the very overlapping symptoms that he had observed in 1,200 cases—mostly women—in his database of aspartame toxicity.

In his book, *Breast Implants or Aspartame (NutraSweet®) Disease?* (ISBN 1-884243-10-X), Dr. Roberts identifies health problems such as headaches, dizziness, confusion, memory loss—Alzheimer's disease—seizures, insomnia, chronic fatigue, hypoglycemia, joint pains, hair loss and rashes as reproducible problems that can be caused by aspartame. He has written a number of other articles and books on this topic.

In a widely circulated article by Nancy Markle, she states that even the Gulf War Veterans' Syndrome of ill health can be blamed on aspartame toxicity caused by the exposure of diet soda supplies in the military camps to the excessive heat of the desert. Heat above 86 degrees F can cause decomposition of the sweetener and produce the neurotoxic elements, methyl-alcohol, formaldehyde and formic acid. The heat in the desert in Saudi Arabia and Kuwait regularly reaches around 130 degrees F.

Those of you who have read my book, *Your Body's Many Cries for Water,* or have listened to my lectures know that I too have been a very strong opponent of the use of artificial sweeteners for the same reason. Remember, artificial sweeteners, aspartame in particular, are dangerous. They can cause a host of disease conditions, including cancer of the bladder, breast, and possibly prostate, as well as brain tumors. Do not take this statement lightly.

Postscript

Below is my *brief* interpretation of an article by Jens Jordan, M.D., and associates for application of their findings to the topics under discussion here. I had to create space in this book, which was already completed and typeset for publication, to share the benefits of this research on water with my readers.

Scientific Explanation for the Medicinal Value of Water in Asthma, Allergies and Lupus

New research by Jens Jordan, M.D., and ten of his medical associates, published in the *Journal of Circulation*, February 2000, has revealed an important direct relationship between water consumption and sustained activation of the sympathetic nervous system and adrenaline production in the body. They discovered that within five minutes of drinking 250 to 450 ccs. (about 8-16 ounces) of ordinary tap water the adrenaline-producing nerve systems are stimulated for more than 90 minutes.

This research reveals exact scientific reasons for the effect of water in the cure of asthma, allergies and lupus. These reasons are, one, when water by itself activates adrenaline production, in effect it directs the body toward physical activity and tissue reconstruction; and, two, water reverses the impact of dehydration and its associated drastic tissue breakdown that is fundamental to eventual disease production in the body.

By its sustained activation of the adrenergic nerve system, water acts as a natural inhibitor of histamine's overactivity. As you now know, histamine is responsible for the drought management programs of the body. The local or regional manifestations of drought have until now been labeled as "diseases" such as asthma, allergies, lupus, adult-onset diabetes, and other autoimmune diseases. Thus, water is an ideal preventive medication in these conditions.

By activating the adrenergic system in the body, within five minutes of intake, water also exposes its superior emergency medicinal value in severe asthma attacks. The patient can achieve natural relief without urgently needing to go to hospital. In hospital, the suffocating asthmatic would only receive an intravenous saline solution, oxygen and an injection of adrenaline. Adrenaline is a very potent antihistamine. It aborts asthma attacks. However, water causes a natural and sustained, *cost-free* release of adrenaline by the nerve systems of the body itself, long before the "suffocating stage" of an asthma attack can develop. Additionally, the use of water in asthma is danger-free, whereas the use of adrenaline for the treatment of severe shortness of breath can sometimes cause death, particularly if the attending physician confuses bronchial asthma with the shortness of breath caused by heart problems.

When the adrenergic system is activated and adrenaline secretion ensues, certain enzyme systems that regulate body metabolism are also stimulated into activity. One of these enzyme systems involves the activation of a fat-breaking and -burning enzyme called "hormone-sensitive lipase." This enzyme initiates the release of energy from the fat stores in the body and decreases the need to break down muscles and protein reserves of the body for energy conversion. In short, through its sustained activation of the adrenaline-secreting nerve system and its action on other metabolic pathways, water prevents "cannibalistic" attacks on the tissues of the body itself and promotes a more "constructive" metabolism in the body—an ideal first step in the treatment of lupus.

During its presence in blood circulation, hormone-sensitive lipase also acts on cholesterol plaques and causes them to shrink and eventually disappear. Thus, water by itself is the best natural anticholesterol medication. Cholesterol-lowering chemical medications are dangerous. They can cause allergies and autoimmune reactions in the liver that can lead to irreversible damage and death.

It seems that when water by itself enters the body, it can raise blood pressure; however, if salt is made available to the body, the rise in blood pressure is not significant. This research finding proves my view that salt is essential for the body and it has a definite *"blood pressure-lowering and heart-calming effect,"* contrary to presently held views in medicine. Strict attention to daily salt intake is vital for prevention of heart damage that can be caused by continuous stimulation of the sympathetic nerve system when *only* water is taken.

Other Qualities of Drinking Water

Water should be clear of toxic metals and bacterial and parasitic contamination. Unfortunately, in industrial countries, the devastating effect of pouring chemical and toxic waste in rivers and lakes is not fully appreciated. As a result of this careless indifference, many of the sources of drinking water have become contaminated. This problem is compounded by the age of water pipes that were laid in urban areas many decades ago. They have by now collected layers of deposit. Further problems are caused by the age and inadequacies of water filtration and treatment plants that are not equal to the present-day demands of some major cities. Several cities are now addressing this problem.

Although chlorination of water is adequate against bacterial and amebic contaminants at the lower, normal and acceptable levels of chlorine, it is not fully effective against heavy contamination by cryptosporidia and, possibly, giardia. These parasites can cause health problems in some people with naturally suppressed immune systems, if the water is heavily contaminated. Fortunately, cryptosporidia seem to be a problem only when there is a lot of rain. Surface water after heavy rains carries large quantities of these animal parasites from the pasture fields to the rivers that are the source of drinking water for major cities. Such rises in contamination necessitate adjustments to the level of chlorination of the water.

This problem of parasite contamination of water achieved national exposure several years ago when it affected some parts of Minnesota, the city of Washington, DC., and parts of northern Virginia where I live. This problem arose from inefficient testing procedures. The water authorities are now more careful, and test the water supply system more often and much more carefully. The problem seems to pose less of a danger than has been presented in the media, which seem to benefit from scaring people.

It seems that cryptosporidia can only cause ill health in people whose immune systems are not functioning well; otherwise the immune system in the human body can easily kill and dispose of the parasites in normal circumstances.

Fluoridation and chlorination of water are two hot issues. Fluoride is added to water to prevent dental decay in children. There is a movement afoot to stop fluoridation of water because it is being blamed for teeth and gum deformity in some people. It is also classified as a potential carcinogen. Opposing this view are some scientists who have shown fluoride helps to increase bone density in people with osteoporosis. In recent molecular research on fluoride intake by the cells of the body, it was shown that fluoride is only picked up by cells that are already damaged. Normally functioning cells do not concentrate fluoride inside them. This research indicates that it is not fluoride that causes cell damage and that the interior cell concentration of fluoride is a postdamage event.

Chlorine seems to be offensive to most people for its smell and taste in water. Please bear in mind that chlorine and its bacteria-killing action is the greatest gift to us who live in these times. Without chlorine, people would die in their millions from devastating infections such as cholera, salmonella, and many more. You need to think about chlorine with gratitude. If you find its smell bothersome, let the water stand for a half hour in an open-top jug. Since chlorine is a natural gas, it will evaporate and the water will become sweet and will not smell. Basically, if you are sensitive to the smell of chlorine, you should not drink water directly from the tap without letting it first stand a while. This is how restaurants serve water: by letting it stand in jugs before they serve it. You can easily and safely drink this water without having to pay for brand-name water. You should not let your body go without water because of the level of chlorine it contains. You can get rid of the chlorine very easily.

Paul Gonzalez is a radio talk show host with United Broadcast Network that airs his show from 110 radio stations across America and also through the Internet to the world. I have been on his show many times. During one of my interviews, on

November 30, 1998, Mr. Gonzalez announced the result of an experiment he conducted with tap water, an experiment that I had suggested in my *Cries for Water* book. He let tap water stand for a while in a jug. He then collected some empty "designer" water bottles, filled them with the tap water, and offered this water to his visitors. Without exception, his friends were complimentary about the taste of the bottled water. When he told them they were drinking ordinary tap water that had been left to stand for a short while, none of them could believe it. They could not imagine how easily the chlorine smell had been cleared, leaving the water tasting clean and "sweet."

The high mineral content of water should not be an issue. If the water contains more of the mineral calcium, it might be more of a help than you think—it is a good source of already dissolved calcium. Research has shown that a high calcium content in drinking water does not necessarily cause more stones in the kidneys.

In the not-too-distant future, I predict most homes will be equipped with a home water filter unit. It will not be practical for local governments to provide 100 percent high-quality drinking water through municipal water systems when no more than 5 percent of that water is used for drinking and cooking purposes. They will begin to legislate for lower standards of the water quality that will be provided to consumers at a much higher cost than today.

If you are concerned about the quality of water in your area, and there is a possibility that it might contain toxic metals such as lead, mercury, cadmium, and too much iron or aluminum, you should get an alternative source of supply. A prudent alternative is to attach a solid carbon filter to the faucet in your kitchen. After the initial cost of about $150 for the filter unit, it should cost no more than $35 a year to change the carbon cartridge. Each carbon filter unit can produce more than 600 gallons of high-quality drinking water, so each gallon of water will cost less than eight cents. By having your own source of high-quality, safe drinking water, your body will not become dehydrated because you do not like the taste of tap water. Solid carbon filters remove all the toxic metals, chemicals, chlorine, some fluoride, bacteria, giardia and cryptosporidia.

People have often asked me what sort of water filter they should use. Normally, I do not make recommendations on products unless a unique situation arises that is to the benefit of people who have trust in me and my words.

Recently I came across a special type of water filter manufactured by NRG Water Products that uses a filter unit made of a layer of solid carbon and a core layer of ceramic. Ceramic is normally used in laboratory filter units that have to produce water of the utmost purity. The combination of carbon and ceramic is most effective against toxic metals, bacteria, parasites and chemical pollutants of water.

Although the company is a wholesaler and does not get involved in the retail sale of its products, I have negotiated with them to sell their products to my readers at a substantial discount.

"Sterling Spring Gold" filters are designed for either under the sink connection or for countertop use. They have a useful electronic metering system that indicates when the cartridge needs to be changed. The units sell for between $200 and $300, depending on the agent and the location of the sale. However, they have agreed to sell these units to my readers at $125 each. In addition, they have also agreed to allocate some funds to be spent on the dissemination of my information on chronic, unintentional dehydration. To order the unit of your choice or its core cartridge, call 1-800-256-0417, and ask for Dr. Batman's special discount.

Let me remind you, only in some parts of the country is the use of a filter desirable. You should check with your local water supplier as to the quality of water in your area.

If you have a well, no matter how sure you are of the quality of the water, you should have it tested frequently. Chlorinate it every so often to prevent bacterial and fungal growth in the stagnant water. You should routinely check the casing of your well for surface-water leaks into the well. Surface-water seepage into the well could contaminate your water with animal parasites. A great offender is giardia.

For washing purposes, and to prevent chlorine burns on your skin, it is advisable to attach a chlorine filter to the shower head in the bathroom. *Water from such a filter is not safe to drink.*

In Summary. The best daily program *to become radiantly well and vibrantly alive* is as follows. Drink sufficient water to achieve a colorless urine. Take enough salt to balance the natural osmotic forces and generate hydroelectric energy for all cell functions in the body. Make sure you use your muscles enough to regulate the chemistry of your brain. Eat a balanced diet that contains high protein and green leafy vegetables. Eat less sugar and fewer starchy foods that convert to fat unless you burn them by intense muscle activity. Avoid alcoholic or caffeine-containing beverages and sodas. This is the only way to remain healthy. Drink at least two glasses of water first thing in the morning to offset the imperceptible water loss you have had during eight hours of sleep (Figure 17).

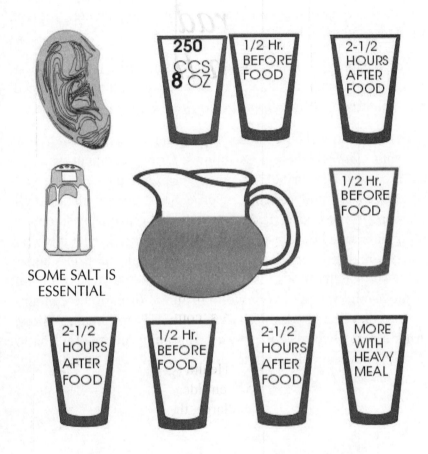

SOME SALT IS
ESSENTIAL

WATER SHOULD BE TAKEN **BEFORE FOOD**
TO PREVENT BLOOD CONCENTRATION

Figure 17

10

Asthma Eradication: It's History in the Making

Asthma: Fraud and Sting Against the Public

The sick care system thrives on the sick remaining sick and ignorant of the natural causes of their health problems. The sick care system in America is composed of the following institutions:

1) The National Institutes of Health (NIH) that spend over $10 billion a year researching different ideas about the conditions of ill health in our society. By and large, they promote "better drug" treatments.

2) The AMA that has many hundreds of thousands of doctors as its members and had, until recently, controlled the way that medical doctors should think and treat their patients. The AMA still cannot tolerate free thinkers and medical mavericks, even if their patients are being cured of their problems. The AMA still organizes the process of removing these doctors' licenses to practice.

3) The HMOs and the insurance companies that regularly hike their prices, yet cover and deliver less and less.

4) The pharmaceutical industry that has maliciously deviated medicine from its physiology-based research and has created the *art of dispensing chemical palliatives for temporary relief and protracted treatment protocols.* The medical profession has unwittingly also bought into this policy, because it is financially a more dependable approach.

5) The fund-raising national foundations that take sob stories to the public and collect money for more research of the same through their favorite research institutes or hospitals. They almost always have people from the AMA on their staff and boards of directors that will shoot any "unorthodox" idea off the discussion table.

6) Last, but most potent of them all, the media that take vast sums of money from the sick care system advertisers and hype their message into the minds of the public. In the words of a highly visible news anchor, "... not biting the hands that feed them."

I have detailed my dealings with the NIH and the AMA, and their obstructive disinterest in chronic dehydration as the origin of the prevalent health problems of the public, in my book, *Your Body's Many Cries for Water.* If you have already read this book, you know how hard, yet naively, I tried to get these trusted national icons of medicine to take a serious look at water as the medication of choice in the health problems I listed at the beginning of this book. I will not waste your time by discussing HMOs and the insurance industry here. You all know about their mode of operation. Here I will expose the other sectors within the sick care system.

Why I Think the Drug Companies Are Not Truthful

As I have described in *Your Body's Many Cries for Water,* I have the scientific distinction of having successfully treated with only water more than 3,000 people suffering from peptic ulcer disease. My report of this success was published as the main editorial of the *Journal of Clinical Gastroenterology* in June 1983, and was also reported in the SCIENCE WATCH (Science Times) of the *New York Times*, June 21, 1983.

To me as a clinician, it became obvious that the people I treated with water were suffering from a "thirst problem," and the label of "disease" is something we have concocted because we have not understood that pain and local damage can be one of the ways that persistent drought in the body shows itself.

One day, at a meeting held in the office of Professor Howard Spiro of Yale University, I made this view known. Professor Gregory Eastwood, who was then head of the Department of Gastroenterology at the University of Massachusetts, and who is now dean of a prestigious medical school, asked me if I could prove this view scientifically. I said I could.

I set out to scientifically prove the view that the human body can produce pain when it is thirsty—and I did it simply!

Drug companies manufacture a class of chemicals that are strong antihistamines. As you know by now, histamine is a brain chemical—a neurotransmitter—whose action the drug industry is determined to block when there is pain. Most strong pain medications are antihistamines. There are many kinds produced by different companies. One variety is Tagamet, another is Zantac. These two are now nonprescription drugs that you can buy off the shelf.

I set out to research why histamine is the target when pain medications are used. Bingo! I discovered that histamine is a vital chemical messenger in the brain. Histamine has a most important function not written about in medical textbooks. As you have learned, it is in charge of water intake and drought management in the body. It is less active when the body is fully hydrated and becomes increasingly active when the body becomes dehydrated. This was the connection I was looking for.

In short, histamine produces pain when an area in the body is suffering from drought!

I had to search through numerous scientific journals to collect this information. It took several months to put this information together. I made several copies of a thick scientific volume and had each volume bound—in April 1985, 15 years ago! A copy was sent to each of the professors who was present at the meeting in Professor Spiro's office.

I subsequently presented at various conferences the discovery that the human body produces pain and develops various diseases when it is suffering from drought. One such conference was the 3rd Interscience World Conference on Inflammation, held in Monte Carlo in 1989. I was invited to make this presentation because, in 1987 as the guest lecturer at an internationally convened conference of selected cancer researchers, I had first revealed this action of histamine while I was explaining that cancer is one of the outcomes of chronic dehydration. The text of my presentation was published in the *Journal of Anticancer Research* in Sept.-Oct. 1987. The abstract of my presentation at the 3rd Interscience World Conference is printed on page 37 of the book of abstracts of the conference, and on page 104 of this book.

Deception and Human Suffering!

Here is a story that should dispel any myths about drug companies being on the side of consumers. In the autumn of 1988, I was asked to speak at the Gastroenterology Society meeting held at the Armed Forces Hospital in Riyadh, Saudi Arabia—a hospital and a country that lack nothing money can buy. I was introduced to the local representative of a major drug company that manufactures one of these special antihistamine pain medications. He did not know me or the topic of my presentation. He was curious. Here I was in Saudi Arabia, from America, addressing a medical gathering.

He asked me, "Do you use our product?" I answered, "No, I do not." He asked, " Are you using the product of our competitor?" I said, "No, I do not use the product of your competitor either."

With much surprise he asked, "Then, what do you use to treat your patients?" I told him, "I use water." In amazement, he said, "What, water alone?" "Yes," I said, "Water alone."

Then I asked him the two questions that had bothered me for some time. "As a researcher into the effect of histamine functions on the body physiology, your company must be aware of the primary role of histamine in water regulation and drought management of the body. Firstly, why do you insist that its actions should be blocked? And, secondly, why do you not explain this water-regulatory role of histamine in the body to the clinicians who are being asked to block its action by the use of your product?"

What do you think his answer was? In an irritated tone of voice, he replied, "We are not here to educate the doctors. They should discover that for themselves! We are a manufacturing company interested in selling a product."

Exactly what I expected! Fortunately, I am now able to reveal what drug companies have been concealing for years from doctors and their patients. It is obvious these companies understand the intricate actions of histamine in the body or else they would not be able to produce specific chemicals that block the union of histamine with its receiving point on the cell membrane. They know that the primary functions of histamine are energy regulation and drought management in the body. They know that water is a better natural antihistamine. Unfortunately, they have also learned how to conceal this information and not let it get into the textbooks of medicine and physiology.

The new knowledge you now possess will make the practice of medicine much simpler and friendlier to you, your health, and your financial resources. What is more, medical jargon will no longer get in your way of understanding your own body and its ways of talking to you. What you need to learn is that water is a safe, natural antihistamine that the body is calling for any time it manifests a health problem.

11

Your Charity! Whose Pork?

The Asthma and Allergy Foundation of America and I

Mr. Paul Harvey of Paul Harvey ABC News had, without prompting, read my book and announced the gist of my findings in one of his news programs. He also wrote a syndicated column that was published in over 200 newspapers across America. When I discovered him to be sympathetic to my crusade, from time to time I sent him more information. On one occasion I sent him information on asthma being curable by water and that millions of children suffer from this problem, and many thousands die each year, not knowing that they are only dehydrated. He then let his audience know that asthmatics should drink more water—a simple public health announcement.

Paul Harvey is a legend and has many followers. Some among his audience happened to be donors to the Los Angeles Chapter of the Asthma and Allergy Foundation of America. They bombarded the Foundation with telephone calls and requests to follow up on this new discovery. Mrs. Francine Lifson, the Foundation's President, called me and asked if what Paul Harvey News had reported was true. I assured her it was. She asked if anyone had been cured from asthma just by drinking water, and asked if I could I send her more information. I told her that quite a number of asthmatics had been cured by water. I immediately faxed her the letter that appears below, along with nine pages of supporting information.

Attention Ms. Francine Lifson
Executive Director
Asthma and Allergy Foundation of America,
Los Angeles Chapter
June 6, 1995

Dear Ms. Lifson:

This must be a historic moment for you and your Foundation that you get the good news that at last asthma has been shown to have a very easy and simple cure.

The enclosed materials verify the fact that people have been cured by the increased intake of water and some salt. For more information, you need to read my book, Your Body's Many Cries for Water.

The abstract of my presentation on the neurotransmitter histamine will show that my approach to the treatment of asthma and allergy has solid scientific basis.

> *Sincerely,*
> *F. Batmanghelidj*

🐦 🐦 🐦 🐦 🐦

The next day, I wrote to Ms. Lifson again and sent her a copy of my book, *Your Body's Many Cries for Water*. I called her a few times during the weeks that followed. At first, I was blocked by the telephone operator. When eventually I spoke to her again, she promised to take a look at the materials I had sent. In the two and a half months that I pursued the matter, I realized she was evading the issue. Eventually she said that the medical doctor on their Board would get in touch with me. He never did. I wrote to her again on September 19, 1995. The letter printed below tells the story.

Ms. Francine Lifson
Executive Director
Asthma and Allergy Foundation of America
Los Angeles Chapter
5225 Wilshire Boulevard, Suite 705
Los Angeles, CA 90036-4216
September 7, 1995

"End of Asthma in Five Years Project"

Dear Ms. Lifson:

Let me summarize: I responded to your enthusiastic inquiry when you received repeated calls from your local residents after the Paul Harvey News announcement on June 5 of a cure for asthma with increased water intake. During our telephone conversations on June 6 and 7, you asked me, "Has anyone been cured of asthma by increased water intake?" I assured you that water does cure asthma and that increased water intake is the natural way to prevent and cure the problem. I then sent you adequate information in the form of reviews, articles, the abstract of the new scientific information on the water regulatory roles of the neurotransmitter histamine, in addition to the book, Your Body's Many Cries for Water. This information revealed to you my discovery that <u>asthma is one of a variety of emergency manifestations of chronic dehydration in the human body</u>.

I was under the impression that you would be genuinely interested in the discovery that a simple cure for asthma is now available. When I did not hear from you, I called you a number of times before I could speak to you. You seemed to be in meetings most of the time. When we spoke the first time, you indicated that

*you did not yet have the time to take a serious look at the infor-
mation. I called you a second time. This time you indicated that
you were short-handed and your office was about to relocate and
you were not able to spend the time to read what I had sent you.
You promised to take the materials home, make the effort to study
them, and get back to me soon. When I did not hear from you
after a few weeks, I called a third time. This time you told me you
had read all of what I had sent you. However, you said: "It is too
simple. I don't believe it." You also told me your consultant physician said asthma was an inflammatory process.*

*I indicated to you that it is true that asthma is the outcome of
an inflammatory process; however, the main cause of the inflammation is water shortage in the body. I explained that, in dehydration, "histamine" becomes active as the main drought man-
ager. It is histamine that causes the inflammation and constriction of the bronchioles—to prevent the lung tissue from drying up
and to reduce the evaporation of water during respiration. I said
I had sent you a copy of the abstract of my presentation on histamine at the 3rd Interscience World Conference On
Inflammation in March of 1989 in order to stress the scientific
basis of my statements.*

*It seemed during our conversation that you had become "hos-
tile" to the new understanding that asthma is a complication of
dehydration and that water can cure it. It was then that I told you
that, now we know the origin of the disease, it would not be
morally correct to go to the public and ask for donations to do
more research along the same lines as before. I asked you for the
names of the members on your Board of Directors so that I could
inform them directly of the scientific breakthrough in the treatment of asthma. You resisted releasing their names and said that
I should send the information to you. I told you that you were
already in possession of the information and should report it to
your Board. When you realized that the news of your refusal to
take the information to your supporters may become a public*

*issue, you offered to get your medical consultant to contact me.
He never did.*

*It is therefore your apparent insensitivity to the fears, the
forced limitations, anguish of those who suffer the devastations
and eventually irreparable damage of chronic dehydration, that
has forced me to take this course. Some of these asthmatics are
innocent children who not only suffer from the constant fear of
choking to death, but will eventually suffer from irreversible
genetic damage because of dehydration. Your unilateral refusal
to engage your Foundation in dealing with this new science of
physiology-based prevention and cure of asthma leaves many
people vulnerable. Those who donate money for research need to
be informed that a solution is now available and will become
part of the research program of the Foundation. The people who
come to you for guidance should also be given educational
pieces that reflect the new information.*

*Any action short of these steps would reflect a betrayal of pub-
lic trust. It would be contrary to the spirit and the laws govern-
ing the existence of philanthropic institutions that depend on
charitable donations. Naturally, the primary purpose of charitable contributions is to serve the purpose for which money is
being collected, and not the creation and maintenance of the
institutions themselves.*

*I invite you to pay serious attention to and rethink your atti-
tude towards the discovery that asthma is a complication of
chronic dehydration. You or your advisors cannot brush aside
this information just because you feel like it. Be so kind as to
send a copy of this letter to every member of your Board of
Directors for their information.*

*A copy of this letter and the pertinent information you have
already received are being sent to the Attorney General of the*

United States, who is the public trustee for all charitable organ-
izations, and the media listed below.

Sincerely,

F. Batmanghelidj

Copy to: Attorney General of the United States
Paul Harvey News
Los Angeles Times
USA TODAY

☞ ☞ ☞ ☞ ☞

I realized that this fund-raising front for the sick care system
was not genuinely interested in finding a natural and permanent
cure for asthma. It would be counterproductive to its very survival. The Foundation is very happy with the theatrics within the
status quo.

I wrote to the Attorney General and enclosed the Lifson
letter.

The Honorable Janet Reno
Attorney General of United States
Department of Justice—Room 4400
Tenth and Constitution Avenue, NW
Washington DC 20530
22 September 1995

Dear Madam Attorney General:

On behalf of millions of children, 12 million of them
Americans, I beg for your attention.

The enclosed information explains the medical discovery that
the human body has a number of emergency reactions to chronic dehydration. The medical community, not being aware of the
regional manifestations of the body to its water shortage, has
traditionally been taught to treat the different symptoms and

signs of dehydration with chemical products or invasive proce-dures. Thus: the health crisis of the American nation.

I am a medical doctor and have done clinical and scientific research on the role of water in disease prevention over the past 15 years. I have proven that many of the prevalent degenerative diseases of the human body are no more than the complications of chronic dehydration. This simple discovery exposes an extremely cost-effective way of prevention and cure to many of today's diseases. The book, "Your Body's Many Cries for Water," explains in greater detail why persistent dehydration causes the conditions that are labeled as diseases of unknown cause.

One of the many conditions that are produced as a complica-tion of dehydration is asthma. This problem is extremely devas-tating to the children who are in the process of growth and need water to develop. If you peruse the pages 114-122 in the book and view the copy of WYOU TV 22—CBS News, THE WATER CURE, you will see that asthma can now be cured very easily.

As the copy of my letter to Ms. Lifson, the Executive Director of the Asthma and Allergy Foundation of America, Chapter of Los Angeles (attached) shows, I have come up against a brick wall in trying to communicate this information for its evaluation and dissemination. The executive director has chosen to ignore my findings and refused to pass them on to her Board of Directors, saying my discovery is "too simple to be believed."

I appeal to you as the chief authority in charge of charitable foundations that collect money, particularly for medical research, for investigation of why the above Foundation refuses to engage in the study of chronic dehydration as the cause of asthma. Surely, if water is simply the ultimate medicine, why not use it! I hope you appreciate that commercial institutions will not fund research that would simplify treatment procedures in medicine.

> Respectfully yours,
> F. Batmanghelidj

Attachments and enclosures:

☞ ☞ ☞ ☞ ☞

I also sent the same letter to the Deputy Attorney General, The Honorable Jamie Gorelick, on October 30, 1995 and started her letter by pleading:

On 22 September 1995, I sent an appeal to the Attorney General. The urgency of my appeal is such that it compels me to present it to you as well. I hope one of you will take my alarm seriously and act upon it.

☞ ☞ ☞ ☞ ☞

I must say in fairness to Ms. Gorelick that one of her assistants, Dennis M. Corrigan, wrote me a letter and told me that the Attorney General's office was not in a position to comment on scientific matters. He advised me to contact Dr. William Harlan, the Director of the Office of Disease Prevention at the NIH.

Obviously they had misunderstood the main reason for my communicating with the Office of the Attorney General. I was complaining about the Asthma and Allergy Foundation's practice of collecting money under the guise of seeking a cure for asthma. Now that the science-based and tested cure is available for them to disseminate, they do not engage in its evaluation lest it prove their undoing.

As a matter of fact, I did write to Dr. Harlan and sent him my book. I said: *"When you read the book, you will see that I have gone the NIH route—without success. However, if the new information on dehydration appeals to your sense of logic and com-*

mon sense, and you wish to actively explore the new possibilities it offers, please be so gracious as to give me a call."

He never got back to me! I knew he would not!

For its historic value, here is the letter from Mr. Corrigan, and my reply, for you to see how far I have gone to get my God-given discovery to the American people through the normal channels— channels that you fund and keep alive with your tax dollars. You give them your vote to get elected, you pay their salaries, but they serve the people who fund their advertising programs just to be elected. Their promise and the oath to serve you become sub-servient to the motives of their cash-for-election benefactors.

U.S. Department of Justice

Office of the Deputy Attorney General

_____

Washington, DC 20530

November 14, 1995

Dr. Fereydoon Batmanghelidj
2146 Kings Garden Way
Falls Church, Virginia   22043

Dear Dr. Batmanghelidj:

    The Deputy Attorney General has referred your letter to me
for response. As you may be aware, the Department of Justice is
not designated to evaluate proposed medical remedies, such as the
one described in your letter.

    By copy of this letter, I am therefore referring your
request to the office of Dr. William R. Harlan, who is the
Director of the Office of Disease Prevention at the National
Institute of Health.

                              Sincerely,

                              Dennis M. Corrigan
                              Executive Assistant and
                                Counsel to the
                                Deputy Attorney General

cc: Dr. William Harlan

Fereydoon Batmanghelidj, M.D.

2146 KINGS GARDEN WAY • FALLS CHURCH • VA 22043 • U.S.A.
Telephone 703 448 7524 - 703 848 2333 - 703 848 2332 • FAX 703 848 2334

Dennis M. Corrigan
Executive Assistant and Counsel
to the Deputy Attorney General
U.S. Department of Justice
Office of the Deputy Attorney General
Washington, DC 20530   November 16, 1995

Dear Mr. Corrigan:

Thank you for your letter of November 14 and the referral to Dr. William Harlan of the NIH.

I do know that the Department of Justice is not in a position to evaluate medical remedies. I was, however, under the impression the Department was in a position to question why a publicly funded Foundation ignored a simple and costless solution to asthma, a devastating breathing problem that affects 12,000,000 children, and kills quite a number each year.

I doubt the benefits of the new information on chronic dehydration as a symptom- and disease-producing state of the body will reach the public through the NIH or the AMA any time soon. The preface of my book will show I have tried these routes before. However, I will contact Dr. Harlan now that you have referred me to him.

In any event, and for future commentary, it is now on record that I had to resort to the Justice Department in my attempt to change the established medical thinking in America.

I have pleasure in seding you a copy of my water book for your personal reading.

Sincerely

F. Batmanghelidj
Enclosure:

Support Groups in the Sick Care System

Another component of the sick care system are the support groups that are created to enforce the dominance of the status quo. On page 197 is the letter Connie Giblin wrote to the editor of her local newspaper, *The Times Leader*, in Wilkes-Barre, PA, on February 21, 1997. Connie has seen how asthma and allergies can be cured by an upward adjustment of daily water intake. She wanted to share this discovery with local asthmatics that gather together for affirmation and support, but she was not allowed to spread her information.

Thus, another group of players operating within the sick care system is exposed. Their malicious perpetuation of ignorance about asthma is to their own advantage, for the benefit of maintaining their position, power and money, without regard to the fact that the health of millions of people is at stake and many thousands die as a result every year.

When concerned persons pledge themselves to helping people in need, they become altruistic and unselfish to the nth degree. Bob Butts, of Wilkes-Barre, PA, is one such champion. He has spent more than $300,000 of his own money to help people understand the health and wellness miracle of the *water cure*. One of his obstacle-removing actions to help asthmatics was his idea of an "asthma billboard." Figure 18 on page 198 is a picture of the billboard that saved many asthmatics from the agony of their affliction.

Mail Bag

The Times Leader, Wilkes-Barre, PA, Friday, February 21, 1997

Hope through the 'water cure' withheld from asthma support group

Editor:

I recently attended the first Asthma Support Group sponsored by a Pennsylvania rehabilitation center on Jan. 27.

I was there with Bob Butts, promoter of the "water cure," and an asthmatic named Sandy.

Tony, one of the therapists, told us how the "water cure" by Dr. F. Batmanghelidj helped his asthma and recommended it to everyone there.

Everyone said they had heard the radio spots and saw the newspaper ads on the "water cure." But I was sad to see one of the facilitators cut Tony's talk short.

Bob was then given permission to speak, but was immediately stopped and rudely told that this was not the place and time to discuss the "water cure," but that they would consider having Bob as a future speaker. That was a joke because Bob was later told not to give out any information on the "water cure" on the premises.

I thought to myself, "This is a support group?"

I guess when you are selling rehab to asthmatics, the last thing anyone wants to hear is something that will make their jobs unnecessary.

Then it was Sandy's turn to talk. She mentioned how the "water cure" reduced her asthma, cutting it by 90 percent. But she was cut short also.

Then it was my turn. I said I never had asthma, but did suffer from bronchitis and severe allergies which according to Dr. Batmanghelidj go hand-in-hand. I have been cured of all my allergies and bronchitis. They didn't want to hear that. And once again we were told, "You don't belong here."

They were right. We didn't belong there because we don't support asthma, we support its cure: the "water cure."

All wrong is done out of ignorance. I truly believe after attending this support group that its sponsors are ignorant.

Is it also possible that they are only interested in keeping people sick for profit? It appears that there is a ton of money being made on rehab, and the "water cure" is a big threat to this profit bonanza.

But we'll win because we work from the heart, not from the wallet.

I was not only angered by the attitude of this center, but also felt deeply sorry for all asthmatics out there who will suffer, or possibly die, if they are not told about the "water cure."

Connie Giblin
Kingston

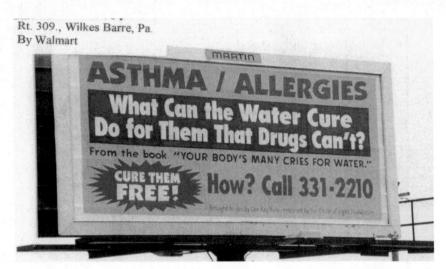

Figure 18

The Media and Their Selective Indifference

From time to time, asthma has become the lead article of one or another of the mainstream media. For the past number of years, I have tried to publish articles about asthma in high-circulation print media. I have tried to get eminent writers and trusted news people to address the issue. I have managed to print my own articles in *Alive* magazine in Canada and have pleaded with Paul Harvey to address the issue in his ABC News program. I am grateful to him for not only voicing the information but also for writing a syndicated column that was published in over 200 newspapers across America. I salute him; he is a discerning friend of his listeners.

I have appeared on many TV shows where I have discussed asthma as a priority. Once I appeared on CNBC's Alive and Wellness program where asthma was the sole topic I discussed for more than 20 minutes. I have been interviewed by radio talk show hosts who have carried my message on dehydration and asthma to many millions of radio listeners all across America. I have tried very hard to meet my deadline of *"An End to Asthma in Five Years."*

I was very touched when, during one of my radio interviews in Pennsylvania, a lady called in to thank me profusely. She said she has two grandchildren who had suffered from severe asthma and she had heard me talk about dehydration and asthma on another radio interview a few months earlier. She had called her daughter and told her that what I said about asthma made sense. They decided to give water a try. The children were given more water and fewer other drinks. Their asthma cleared up. They had been free of their breathing problems and any need for medication for some time when she shared her information with the people who were listening to my radio interview.

Obviously, this message is getting around through my radio interviews, but not fast enough. There are ruthless people and greed-motivated obstacles in the way of more effective dissemination of my natural and physiology-based cure for asthma. It truly upsets me when knowledgeable people in the media choose to ignore this new breakthrough information on asthma. They continue to participate in the spread of money-making, but health-deteriorating, treatment protocols designed to sell more "toxic poisons" to this constantly life-threatened, desperate, anxious, and yet captive sector of our society! Every article the media people write is designed to tighten the sick care industry's grip on the 17 million asthmatics in our society. Every breath these wretched asthmatics take is supposed to make more money for the sick care industry, of which, in my opinion, these media pundits are a part! Let me give you examples.

In its May 1997 issue, *Life* magazine ran a cover story, "Breathe Easy—If you are one of the 50 million Americans with ALLERGIES or ASTHMA, now you can take control of your life." On May 28, 1997, *Newsweek* magazine ran its cover story, "The Scary Spread of Asthma and How to Protect Your Kids." On page 3, there is a picture of a very young child with a breathing mask, and the caption states: "Asthma has shown a huge increase in the past 20 years, particularly among kids. Although new drugs help tame the effect, doctors still haven't figured out the cause of the pandemic." In *Newsweek's* Lifestyle section:

"Asthma is a scary fact of life for millions. Can it be beaten?" by Geoffrey Cowley and Anne Underwood, *Newsweek* gave its views on asthma.

The article begins with the story of 13-year-old Antonio O'Bryant, "who knew the drill by heart." He never went to school without his inhaler full of medication. When he went to his gym class a week before Christmas, he forgot to take his bag with the medication in it. He felt an attack coming. By the time a substitute teacher sent someone for help, and the nurse and an assistant principal got the inhaler to Antonio, he was not breathing enough to get the medication into his lungs. "The nearest hospital was only a mile away, but Antonio was unconscious when he arrived by ambulance." He was in a coma for several days and then his prospects for recovery faded "when his brain started to swell." The ventilator was turned off and Antonio died on Christmas Day.

Every year, thousands of people like Antonio die of exactly the same problem: suffocation from a bad asthma attack. I think science writers like Mr. Geoffrey Cowley—who understand science sufficiently to be able to translate complex discoveries into everyday language for the benefit of the average reader—are also morally responsible for the plight of the 17 million or more asthmatics. In my opinion, they are morally responsible because it seems they put the commercial aims of the news media they work for before the interests of their readers.

They brainwash the public into believing the only way to deal with health problems is to accept the deadly hazards of being "chemically treated" by the sick care system. You see, at the time of writing his article, Mr. Cowley was in possession of ample information on the relationship of asthma and dehydration, and water and histamine. Between 1992—when I first spoke to him on the telephone and sent him a letter and additional information—and 1997, I had written him 10 letters. In August 1993, I wrote him a letter and sent him a copy of my interview with Sam Biser on the subject of asthma. The interview was published in the *Last Chance Health Report Newsletter*. My 21 October 1993 letter to him was again on the topic of asthma. He was also sent a copy of my book and the abstract of my presentation on the neurotransmitter histamine at the 3rd Interscience World Conference on Inflammation *a number of times.*

When he wrote his article, he could have included a discussion of the role of water in the prevention of asthma, which might even have saved Antonio—and thousands like Antonio—from unnecessary and wasteful death. He chose not to and he now stands accused before the court of public opinion for this arrogant and callous disregard of the truth about asthma. Standing accused with him is *Newsweek* magazine which thrives on advertising from the pharmaceutical industry. Every week, it runs many full-page ads that push this or that chemical product. In its May 26, 1997 issue, there were five full-page ads on asthma and allergy medications alone. *Life* magazine's asthma issue ran nine full-page ads on asthma and allergy medications. Thus, the nationally popular mainstream print media use their vast readership and circulation to generate income from the chemical industry that promotes toxic drugs to the media's readers. It is unfortunate that some of these papers go out of their way to obstruct the spread of alternative information that would naturally release some of the sick from the sick care system that has grown into a $1.3 trillion-a-year industry—1998 figures, and rising annually.

Below are some of the letters I wrote to Mr. Cowley of *Newsweek*, inviting him to become part of the science-based solution to asthma. You can see he did not accept my invitation. If you ask him why, he will forget he is a science writer and should understand basic science. He will most probably say water is not yet a proven course of treatment! I have tried the same process with many other science writers who are with major newspapers and magazines. I only use Mr. Cowley as an example because he could have done so much more than others, and he did not. They are all frightened of the final outcome of the information and its impact on the sick care system that they claim to understand and broker.

Attention: Mr. Geoffrey Cowley
Health and Science Editor
Newsweek
444 Madison Avenue
New York, NY 10022
13 August, 1993

Dear Mr. Cowley:

   Further to my letter of 13 April 1993, I have pleasure in send-
ing you a copy of Mr. Sam Biser's Health Newsletter. As you can
see, he has devoted the whole of his newsletter to asthma and the
associated conditions caused by chronic dehydration.

   I also have pleasure in sending you a list of my radio inter-
views and lectures about the water metabolism of the human
body, and its emergency thirst signals, the subject of my book,
"Your Body's Many Cries for Water."

   The medicinal property of water in different "disease condi-
tions" is now exposed. The public will gradually begin to under-
stand that many of the medical conditions that have been given
professional labels of "disease" are no more than indicators of
chronic dehydration—some of the very conditions of unknown
etiology that are discussed in medical textbooks. They will begin
to understand they are not sick. They are only thirsty. As simple
as that! That is when the health care system in America will grad-
ually transform. Not by legislation, but by educating the people
about the simple confusion in medicine that allows different
dehydration-produced conditions of the human body to be treat-
ed with medications or invasive procedures.

   If the solution to many of the health problems of the public is
simply a change in the lifestyle of their fluids intake, is there any
good reason why they should not be given this good news? The
sooner we disseminate this breakthrough information in medi-
cine, the sooner we will be able to cut the health care costs in
America.

I hope the above information will touch a sympathetic chord with your open mind and inner person.

Sincerely,
F. Batmanghelidj

☞ ☞ ☞ ☞ ☞

In October 1993, I again wrote to Mr. Cowley and almost begged him to think seriously and scientifically of dehydration as the primary cause of asthma. Imagine how many thousands of Antonios would have been saved by now. Here is the letter.

Mr. Geoffrey Cowley
21 October 1993

Dear Mr. Cowley:

I REQUEST A FEW MINUTES OF YOUR CLEAR MIND.

- *Do you know what happens to the human body, if it does not receive ADEQUATE water on a regular daily basis?*

- *Do you know what happens to the body if caffeine and alcohol-containing beverages substitute for water, when caffeine and alcohol are known to promote water secretion from the kidneys?*

- *Do you know that a "dry mouth" is not an accurate indicator of water shortage in the human body?*

- *Do you know that the elderly can be seen to have a dry mouth after water deprivation and yet not drink it even if water is made available to them?.*

- *Do you know that between the ages of 20 to 70 the ratio of intracellular water content of the body to its extracellular water content changes from 1.1 and becomes 0.8—less water inside the cells?*

- *Do the cells with less water become independent of the intricate chemical function of water within their cytoplasm and the nucleus?*

- *Do you know that histamine is the main neurotransmitter that regulates water intake and the drought management of the body—that its increased production and release is proportionate to water shortage, particularly in children (histamine is a growth factor)?*

- *Do you know that the human body has a number of very sophisticated emergency thirst signals?*

- *When asthma becomes cured with increased water intake (attachments), are we curing a disease or are we treating a condition produced by extreme dehydration?*

If you do not know the answer to some of these questions, it is time to read about chronic dehydration, a disease-producing state in the human body! When 15,000,000 people suffer from asthma, and several thousands die from it every year, is it fair to them not to know they are not sick, they are only thirsty? In clear conscience and your own personal satisfaction, this is where the power of your pen could make a difference in the lives of millions of people.

Further to our telephone conversation of the 20th, I have pleasure in sending you another copy of my book, "Your Body's Many Cries for Water" and some other pieces of information that complement the statements in the book. We now have the knowledge to transform the health care system and eventually <u>cut its costs by 60 percent</u> in less than ten years. How? By educating the public about emergency thirst signals of the human body! Do you wish to help in this direction?

Sincerely,
F. Batmanghelidj

☞ ☞ ☞ ☞ ☞

I wrote to Mr. Cowley once again on the subject of asthma in 1995. I explained why asthmatics are infinitely more susceptible to other diseases and eventual serious genetic damage. I did not hear from him, nor did he—to my knowledge—write anything on dehydration causing disease. Here is my letter.

Mr. Geoffrey Cowley
30 May, 1995

"END OF ASTHMA IN FIVE YEARS PROJECT"

Dear Mr. Cowley:

The information contained in the enclosed peer-reviewed two books will eventually transform medical knowledge and put it on its future patient-friendly development for the next few hundred years. They explain the etiology of the common degenerative diseases to be chronic dehydration. They explain how to prevent and CURE a variety of diseases that have so far confounded the mainstream medical establishment.

One such CURE is demonstrated for asthma. That is why I have declared: "END OF ASTHMA IN FIVE YEARS." The reason why I am now concentrating on eradication of asthma, as opposed to the cure of the other disease conditions that are also shown in the book, "Your Body's Many Cries for Water," is one simple fact. The bodies of twelve million children who are known to suffer from asthma will not develop normally when they are so dehydrated as to exhibit the outward manifestations of asthma— dehydration and the fourth dimension of time. They will eventually suffer from many other irreparable genetic complications that can be produced by their continued dehydration.

One case in point is Dr. Brown-Christopher, who is an MD herself. Her letter is attached. Dr. Christopher confirms how simply and quickly her son Jeremy has been cured of his devastating asthma. He is now alert, full of energy and enjoys his school much more. His grades have improved significantly. Even his teachers have noticed Jeremy's dramatic change.

The attached confirmations from two medical professionals, as well as the published information that water is a natural anti-histamine, define a simple fact: asthma is a complication of chronic dehydration. Its natural prevention and cure is brought about by constant attention to one's daily water intake. That is all it takes. I invite you to talk to Dr. Brown-Christopher or Dr. Rivera yourself. These are MDs who have first-hand experience about the medicinal properties of water in asthma. They now use the new information about dehydration-produced diseases in their daily practice. You can even talk to Jeremy himself and find out how his life has been changed.

As you see, the information in my book is having a most positive impact on the life of those who come across it. However, it will take too long for this information to reach the parents of some twelve million asthmatic children through the book alone. That is why I am inviting the health news reporters to join me in the spread of information about chronic dehydration as the primary etiology of asthma. Please read the enclosed materials and join me in the honorable crusade of ending asthma in five years. It is emotionally most satisfying to so easily change a constantly suffocating and helpless health situation in young and innocent asthma-suffering children.

> *Sincerely,*
> *F. Batmanghelidj*

Enclosures and attachments

☞ ☞ ☞ ☞ ☞

Bernard Shaw said in 1897: *"The worst sin toward our fellow creatures is not to hate them, but to be indifferent to them: that's the essence of inhumanity."* I think the plight of asthmatics and the lack of enthusiasm on the part of the media to tell them they are only thirsty for water exemplifies Mr. Shaw's views. When I read the 1997 *Newsweek* article, I wrote Mr. Cowley the following letter.

I invited him once again to change his stance of indifference and "perpetuation of medical misinformation" that he had been a party to, and to give his trusting readers a chance. I am writing these lines at the end of February 2000. To date—more than two years later—I have not had a reply from Mr. Cowley. The reason he is featured in this book on asthma is to let the American people know they need to wake up. They are caught in the sick care system sting—and I am a medical doctor writing these words.

Geoffrey Cowley
June 25, 1997

ASTHMA:
CAUSE: Chronic Dehydration
CURE: Water and Salt—Simple, Natural, and Free

Dear Mr. Cowley:

Your asthma article and its perpetuation of the current total misunderstanding and ignorance about this condition has prompted me to write again and remind you that asthma is no longer a "mystery disease." One does not have to become a Sherlock Holmes to deal with this simple problem.

Asthma is simply one of the many different outward manifestations of severe chronic regional dehydration in the human body. Asthma denotes a state of dehydration. The bronchial constriction you have shown in your article, produced by histamine, is a step in the process of drought management. It occurs in order to prevent the free passage of air that would further rob the body of its precious water in the form of vapor through the lungs.

The thick mucus you identified as a problem has two natural purposes: one, to further narrow the air passageways without their having to exert too much energy to contract the muscles to close the lumen. The other, even more important, natural reason for so much mucus is its property of extreme water retention—98 percent—that protects the bronchial epitheliums and prevents their desiccation and peeling off. At the same time, the mucus layer in the bronchioles humidifies the air that goes into the alveoli and prevents excess water loss from the air sac membranes that would otherwise become brittle were they to lose more of their water content than is available to them through the blood circulation.

<u>Water and salt are the best natural elements needed to prevent and cure asthma</u>. They are very strong and effective natural antihistamines. Water will turn off the dehydration-induced excess histamine production, and will also produce the needed surface tension to constrict the alveoli and increase their tidal air exchange. Salt acts as an antihistamine and a natural mucus breaker. Because of its "charge-shielding" property, sodium makes mucus stringy and less sticky—more easily flowing. This medicinal application of water and salt could also be useful in cystic fibrosis.

Now that the cause and a simple natural cure for asthma have been discovered, to permit continued exposure and suffering of millions of dehydrated asthmatics—many millions of them innocent children—to the other irreversible damages of chronic dehydration is cruel and inhuman. It is wrong and immoral to let so many millions live with the constant threat of suffocation and death so that "disease-dependent" medical commerce can continue to thrive the way it is doing now.

The advantage of this discovery is the simplicity of its application. Since chronic dehydration falls into the category of <u>deficiency disorders</u>, its correction is all that is needed to prevent and reverse its major complications—in this case, asthma attacks. One does not need to conduct "double-blind" trials to institute the simple protocol of adjusting daily water and salt intake to prevent and cure asthma. One only needs to discard "prejudices" and take a serious look at its foundation of pure science. The medical breakthrough came about because of the new understanding and explanations of the primary water regulatory functions of histamine—information the drug companies *have possessed all the time, yet have concealed until now. The abstract of my scientific presentation on this aspect of histamine function is attached.*

I hope you will join me in my efforts to eradicate asthma from the list of human sufferings and diseases that are produced by dehydration. At present, they are all lucratively treated with chemical products or "procedures." On my part, I have started to educate the public directly, and am inviting them to join me in this humanitarian cause. My way may take a little longer than if the media participated in this effort, but it is a grassroots approach and will, in the long run, be highly effective.

One such activity is taking place in the region of Scranton and Wilkes-Barre in Pennsylvania. A number of altruistic people in this region, including many chiropractors, have created the Circle of Light Foundation, and are seriously and most effectively engaged in educating the rest of the people in NE Pennsylvania about the health complications of chronic dehydration. On top of their list is asthma. They advertise daily on the radio and television. They have made billboards on the asthma cure. They also generate newspaper articles and ads, and are very active in personal networking. They conduct radio interviews with people who have been cured of asthma. In short, the physiology-based transformation of the "health care system" in America has effectively begun in that part of the world. The "people" are doing it, not the government, the NIH or the AMA; nor are the mainstream media involved. In effect, the "people" are exposing the health care fraud that has been in operation against the American public until now. The newspaper ad challenging the Asthma and Allergy Foundation is attached, as are several other advertisements.

I write this letter to inform you of the new physiology-based medical breakthrough that has exposed the etiology of many "disease" conditions. The new science-based understanding of the origin of many disease conditions happens to benefit the public and not the commercial health care system or the media that depend on its advertising dollars. This is a great moment in the history of humankind. We can now eradicate many disease conditions simply and naturally, and no one can stop this medical truth from spreading. We are starting with asthma because it affects millions of children. You see, the level of dehydration that manifests itself in the form of asthma will also affect the genetic development of the child. We need to protect our future generations from irreversible abnormalities associated with chronic dehydration.

My dear Mr. Cowley, now that we understand what is happening, it would be criminal to remain silent and indifferent to the new medical knowledge in order to protect the status quo. I hope you will begin your own research into what I have just told you, and cause your magazine to become the standard-bearer for the new people-friendly truth in medicine.

> *Yours sincerely,*
> *F. Batmanghelidj, M.D.*

cc: *The Circle of Light Foundation*
Paul Harvey
Dr. Julian Whitaker
Nancy Sander
Life Magazine—Glenn Dowling and Anne Hollister
Asthma and Allergy Foundation of America
Dr. Jonas, the Office of Alternative Medicine, the NIH

Attachments:

☞ ☞ ☞ ☞ ☞

You can now see why basic medical ignorance about dehydration-produced disease—like asthma and allergies—continues; many thousands of Antonios die every year; millions of other asthma and allergy sufferers continue to suffer—all because the sick care industry wants to continue to "carve its pound of flesh" from the body of the unfortunate sector of our society that does not yet know water is an infinitely better medication for many illnesses.

My work does not stop here or with this book. I have hired a lawyer to look into the legal implications and possibilities of starting proceedings against the NIH if they continue to ignore or censor the information about the cure of so many diseases with water. We are identifying asthma as the first line of a "legal invitation."

Where the "Buck" Did Not Stop

Traditionally, they say the buck stops here, when an issue reaches the desk of the President. I heard the President of the United States had allocated millions of dollars to the treatment of asthmatic children. I was touched and I decided to write him a letter and invite him to intervene on behalf of the 12 million children who suffer from asthma and the few thousand of them who die every year.

Bill Clinton
President
The White House
Washington, DC 20500
January 28, 1999

Dear Mr. President:

Today's news has it that you have allocated a substantial amount of money for the study of childhood asthma. What a timely act. Twelve million children suffer from asthma and several thousands suffocate to death from this devastating and deadly scourge of protected medical ignorance.

My dear Mr. President, eradication of the scourge of asthma from our society does not need extensive money- and time-consuming effort, it needs sincerity and scientific integrity to achieve this noble purpose. Scientific information that could bring about this ultimate outcome has been available for some time. It was

even presented at the first Office of Alternative Medicine conference held in Chantilly, 14-16 September, 1992. Needless to say,
the information was censored from the report of the conference
when it was published. Before the OAM conference, the same scientific findings were presented at the 3rd Interscience World
Conference on Inflammation in 1989—the abstract of that presentation is attached.

The enclosed Asthma Special Report makes the now available
science-based natural solution to asthma easy to understand. I
propose that you mandate a priority research of this information
as part of your Presidential Directive. If you project this sincerity of effort, you will see an eradication of asthma from the list of
human diseases in the lifetime of your own Presidency. Should
you choose to champion a study of the wider application of the
topic of the Special Report, history will remember you for the
transformation of medicine that this new scientific discovery
will, sooner or later, bring about, and not what is currently consuming the mind of every member of our society.

Please be so gracious as to inform me of your views and
actions you wish to take.

Respectfully,
F. Batmanghelidj, M.D.

Attachments and enclosures.

☞ ☞ ☞ ☞ ☞

Toward the end of March I received a letter from Claude
Lenfant, M.D., of the NIH. I will transcribe parts of the letter for
your information.

Dear Dr. Batmanghelidj:

Thank you for your letter to President Clinton describing your
interest in asthma treatment and your proposed approach of having patients drink substantial amounts of water. Your letter was

forwarded to me for response as Director of the National Heart, Lung and Blood Institute (NHLBI) .... I am enclosing a copy of the National Asthma Education and Prevention Program's recent Expert Panel Report 2: Guidelines for the Diagnosis and Management of Asthma, which outlines recommendations for asthma therapy based on the review of the published scientific literature.

The advances in our understanding of asthma over the last 20 years have been tremendously exciting and have led to increasingly effective therapy. .... The role of dehydration in initiating the process of histamine release could be a testable hypothesis. There is a growing body of evidence that supports a role for histamine in osmoregulation. However, the significance of osmoregulation in the pathogenesis of asthma has not yet been defined.

.... Furthermore, the NHLBI and the National Institutes of Health's Center for Alternative Medicine work together to support rigorous evaluations of complementary therapies in asthma. If you are interested in learning more about the Center for Alternative Medicine, may I suggest you contact the office at 301-496-4792.

Results from investigations, using randomized, controlled methodologies and published in peer reviewed journals, provide the basis for recommendations in the National Asthma Education and Prevention Program. Continued research in these areas will certainly advance our treatment options.

Thank you again for your interest in asthma.

> *Sincerely yours,*
> *Claude Lenfant, M.D.*
> *Director*

☞ ☞ ☞ ☞ ☞

This letter was a polite brush off. He basically said, *"go stand in line for funding and prove what you want to say according to our way of doing things. We are satisfied with what has been done so far."* I was not satisfied with his protective stance for the status quo. Asthma is afflicting more and more of the younger sector of our society. Dr. Lenfant should claim satisfaction only if the medical establishment can cure the problem without having to prescribe the daily use of an array of inhalers and other medications that devastate the daily life of so many millions of people. I wrote him the the following letter and told him my work is complete and does not need the NIH's approval before it reaches the public. I also posed a poignant question for him to ponder.

Claude Lenfant, M.D.
Director: National Institutes of Health
National Heart, Lung, and Blood Institute
Bethesda, MD 20892
April 2, 1999

> *"A new scientific truth is not usually presented in a way to convince its opponents. Rather they die off, and a rising generation is familiarized with the truth from the start."*
>
> *Max Planck*

Dear Dr. Lenfant:

Thank you for your March 12 response to my letter to President Clinton, and your Expert Panel Report 2 volume. Reading your letter, I was reminded of the Second World War. After World War One, the French thought of preparing their defenses for the next world war that seemed inevitable. They built the Maginot Line, a fortification on their NE border with Germany. They spent much money to create concrete barriers to prevent tanks moving across their border that had been vulnerable in the past. Naturally, the obvious happened. When World War Two broke out, the German army skirted around the constructed defense line and reached Paris in less than a week. The Maginot Line, on which the French had blindly relied, proved inconsequential. It left France most vulnerable because of its reliance on a false assumption that the Germans would try to break through the Line.

Believing incorrectly that dry mouth is the only sign of dehydration in the body, the medical profession has not recognized that most "disease conditions" are really states of dehydration, and their complications. This mistake is the infrastructure of our present "science-based" sick care system. This monster child of ignorance and greed relies upon, and only concentrates on, the development of invasive procedures, or chemical manipulation of the manifestations of dehydration of the human body. It has even constructed its Maginot Line barriers to research for the discovery of physiology-based solutions and cures.

Now comes the new scientific truth: Chronic cellular dehydration of the body is the primary etiology of painful, degenerative diseases. Dehydration can initially reflect its presence by producing pain or by activating the body's drought management programs such as asthma, hypertension, diabetes. All of these indicators of dehydration and its long-term complications are labeled as "diseases of unknown etiology."

Fortunately, this science-based breakthrough information is out in the open and can skirt all barriers and reach the public directly and without hindrance.

To explain myself, I have pleasure in sending you a copy of my book, Your Body's Many Cries for Water, a copy of my video, Cure Pain and Prevent Cancer, and a copy of a half-hour television program, "The Water Cure," produced by a CBS station in Pennsylvania—one of many media programs on the subject—to show how effectively the discovery of the "water cure" is reaching the public directly.

Your comment "the significance of osmoregulation in the pathogenesis of asthma has not yet been defined" brings to attention the vital, natural role of the surface tension of water in producing the uniform contraction of the alveolar membranes in all part of the lungs in order to complete the act of exhaling air. In a state of dehydration, unless histamine increases capillary circulation, to the point of an inflammatory situation, how else is water going to be available for alveolar contraction during routine breathing? This is a question you might choose to answer as guardian of the Heart, Lung, and Blood Institute at the NIH.

People like you need to protect the future of the NIH as the vanguard of advanced medical research and begin to foster the study of the role of water in disease prevention, treatment and cure. Surely, if the NIH continues to disregard the breakthrough information that "dehydration is the primary cause of painful degenerative diseases in the human body," it will become even more irrelevant to the progress of the "new human-applied science of medicine" that is already reaching the public directly?

I do hope you will not take offense at my comments. They are the result of many years of disappointing contacts with the NIH, the AMA, and the Department of Health and Human Services. The preface to my book gives a synopsis of my contacts with your "illustrious" organization. It is unfortunate that the NIH, which is funded by the public, finds it difficult to serve the tax-paying public and commit itself to investigating the new discovery that the human body manifests dehydration in a manner that simulates "disease conditions."

In the light of the new information on dehydration and the human body, it is becoming obvious that—as trusted doctors— we have caused much damage to society and irreversible harm to people. I shudder when I think of the millions of asthmatic children, whose natural cure flows from the faucet of their kitchen, but they receive their doctors' chemical prescriptions! Is this fair? How can we justify so much ignorance? How can we let it continue?

With your permission, I will publish parts of your letter to me, along with this letter and the letter I wrote to President Clinton, in my new book, ABC of Asthma and Allergy, to highlight the con-

tinuing divide between the NIH and the American people. Naturally, it would give me no end of pleasure should you tell me that you have decided to invite proposals from other research centers (my work is completed already) for the study of the effect of water and salt as natural antihistamines in the treatment of asthma, allergies, angina—and any other topic your fiefdom controls. I would naturally announce this most pleasing and popular, positive response as well.

Sincerely,
F. Batmanghelidj, M.D.

Attachments and enclosures:

☞ ☞ ☞ ☞ ☞

I have not had any reply.

You can now see why I have taken an accusatory stance against the mainstream medical establishment and the "people's" elected officials.

Finally

The major disease conditions that humans have to cope with are produced *primarily* by prolonged water shortage in the body. This information has been available to scientists for some time. When this information and the changes it can bring about become common knowledge, the presently recognized major disease problems of mankind, including asthma, allergies and lupus will disappear. Our approach to medicine will become physiological and nature-based, instead of its present pharmacological and toxic-to-the-body-based ways of dealing with health issues. It will become gentle instead of invasive. The vast financial resources of the older and more vulnerable members of society will be freed from fear-driven insurance policies and health expenditures. These people will be able to spend their hard-earned money on more useful and rewarding purposes. Younger people will remain healthy and more productive during a longer life. In short, the life of the individual will become more pleasant and less threatened.

By correcting the explained medical misconceptions on water and salt that have existed up to now, leaps of progress in the science of medicine and a more accurate knowledge of the human body will be its natural rewards.

The public and professionals need to join efforts to make this now-possible change a welcome reality. You cannot sit back thinking that someone else will do it. When people's pain and suffering could be so easily removed, _indifference to this information is the essence of inhumanity_.

Now that our errors of understanding the human body have been exposed, let us walk in humility with our Creator and rise to the high moral ground of becoming the loving and compassionate beings we were meant to be.

About the Author

Dr. Fereydoon Batmanghelidj (pronounced Batman-ge-lij) was born in Iran in 1931. He attended school in Scotland and received his medical training at London University's St. Mary's Hospital Medical School. Upon completion of his studies, he had the privilege of being selected as a house doctor in his own medical school. When he finally returned to Iran to serve the people in his own country, Dr. Batmanghelidj also became engaged in the creation of a sports complex for children, a number of hospitals and his own family charity medical center, the largest medical complex in Iran.

When revolution broke out in 1979, Dr. Batmanghelidj, as a highly visible member of a prominent family, was thrown in jail and all of his and his family's possessions were confiscated. While serving as a political prisoner in Evin prison, he discovered the healing power of water.

One night, Dr. Batmanghelidj had to treat a fellow prisoner who was suffering severe peptic ulcer pain. With no conventional medication at his disposal, Doctor Batmanghelidj gave the man, who was crippled with pain, two glasses of water. Within eight minutes, his pain disappeared. He was instructed to drink two glasses of water every three hours, and he became absolutely pain-free for the four remaining months he was in prison. Without using any medication, the patient was cured.

During the 31 months of his imprisonment, Dr. Batmanghelidj treated more than 3,000 peptic ulcer sufferers with water alone. He conducted extensive research during his prison stay into the medicinal effects of water, and discovered water could prevent, relieve and cure many painful, degenerative diseases. He found Evin prison an "ideal stress laboratory," and chose to stay an extra four months in prison to complete his research into the relationship of dehydration, stress and disease, despite being offered an early release. A report of his findings was smuggled out of

Iran and became the editorial article in the June 1983 issue of the *Journal of Clinical Gastroenterology,* and was also reported on by the *New York Times* Science section.

After his release from prison in 1982, Dr. Batmanghelidj escaped from Iran and came to America, where he continues his research into the role of water in the human body and the damaging effects of dehydration on human health. His studies show that, if we maintain a healthy lifestyle of drinking plenty of water on a regular basis, we will be able to enjoy good health and avoid diseases and painful conditions that require pharmaceutical drugs and expensive medical procedures.

Dr. Batmanghelidj now dedicates his time to promoting public awareness of the healing power of water. His book, *Your Body's Many Cries for Water,* has helped hundreds of thousands of people live happier, healthier lives.

Dr. Batmanghelidj has been a guest on several hundred radio programs and many television shows.

He has written six books. *Your Body's Many Cries for Water,* has been translated into twenty languages. He has also written a special report on pain. His lectures are now available on CD and DVD. The ten hour seminar, *Water RX for a Healthier, Pain-Free Life,* is offered in a CD as well as Audio Cassette format.

****

SOME REVIEWS OF THE
AUTHOR'S PUBLISHED MATERIALS

"One man's solution to soaring health costs: water:"

Paul Harvey

"I was particularly stunned by Dr. Batmanghelidj's lucid description of how lack of water is the primary cause of hypertension, which affects 50 million Americans."

Julian Whitaker, M.D., Health & Healing

"It is claimed that fish probably have no awareness of the presence of water; this book shows we may have done little better. Mostly we have treated symptoms, and often wrongly at that, but masterpieces come into being to produce paradigm shifts. If we learn this one, we may arrest the course of our patients in their all too rapid going the way of all flesh."

Book Reviews, *Journal of Clinical Gastroenterology*

After having read many of Dr. Batmanghelidj's recent works, including his jewel of a book, "Your Body's Many Cries for Water," it is very apparent that this work is revolutionary and sweeps nearly all diseases before it. As an Internist/Cardiologist I find this work incisive, trenchant and fundamental. This work is a God Send for all.

Dan C. Roehm, M.D., F.A.C.P.

"How like 'monkey mind' to bounce about, tying itself in knots with complex solutions while ignoring the profound significance of the simple! Circumstance helped Dr. Batmanghelidj perceive the elegant significance of one factor we too often overlook: water."

Jules Klotter, *Townsend Letter for Doctors*

"Dr. Batman's books are full of common sense and truthful medical advice. His suggested treatment of diseases goes to the roots, the cause of it and anyone who is fortunate enough to read them won't be disappointed with their purchase."

**Laurence A. Malone, M.D., Ph.D.,
Dean for Academic Affairs,
The Learning Center for College Sciences, Ohio**

"I consider your insights some of the most amazing I have encountered in medicine. Sixteen years of private practice in OBG and 8 years as a GP have provided me with a perspective that appreciates the potentials of your proposals."

L. B. Works, M.D., F.A.C.O.G.

"The author, as a result of his extensive clinical and scientific research, concludes that the body possesses many different thirst signals. Many different symptoms and signs of dehydration have until now been viewed as classical diseases of the body."

Frontier Perspectives,
THE CENTER FOR FRONTIER SCIENCES
AT TEMPLE UNIVERSITY

"After many years of study and practicing medicine, it is both rewarding and refreshing to discover the solution to many degenerative conditions beautifully explained by Dr. Batmanghelidj in Your Body's Many Cries for Water. This type of information fills a void left from traditional education."

Robert Battle, M.D.

"Thank you for the timely advice on using the combination of water and salt to treat my asthma. ...not only calmed my coughing but took it away. Once again thank you so much for sharing such insights into complex problems."

Jose A. Rivera, M.D.

"It is a well written book and easy to understand. I think reading of this book should be made compulsory in all the Elementary, Middle and High Schools. It will prevent lots of illnesses and suffering at almost no additional costs."

Hiten Shah, M.D.,
San Jacinto Medical Clinic, CA.

"Batmanghelidj leads us through these entities point by point and weaves a magnificent tapestry if not possibly allopathic medicine's shroud—we can't both be right."

The Biotron Connection

"The Greatest Health Discovery in the World."

Sam Biser,
The University of Natural Healing

"*Batmanghelidj's book Your Body's Many Cries for Water hits the nail on the head period.*"

Arthur Moll, D.C.

"*Dr. Batmanghelidj has researched the phenomenon of pain and water metabolism of the body. His research, published in various scientific journals, has led him to address pain as "proven but seldom recognized signal of local shortage of water in the body."*

The Rotarian

Doctor Finds Ulcer Remedy: "*It started with a patient suffering unbearable ulcer pain one late night. The Doctor treated him with 500 cubic centimeter of water. His pain became less sever and then disappeared completely. The physician was so impressed that he prescribed two glasses of water six times a day and achieved a "clinical" cure of the ulcer attack.*"

The New York Times "Science Watch"

"*When Dr. Batmanghelidj thinks of a glass of water, he doesn't think of it as half full or half empty. He thinks of it as brimming over with the essential fluid of life. He thinks of it as the solvent of of our ills and the deliverer of ripe old age. He thinks of it as the wave of the future.*"

The Washington Times

A Medical Atom Bomb!
"*New! This book by a highly respected M.D. explodes a medical atom bomb—An entirely new paradigm for the cause and prevention of many degenerative diseases! You owe it to yourself to read this incredible book!*"

Nutri-Books

"*The average American is woefully uninformed about water. Most people think they drink enough water, but they don't. Dr. Batmanghelidj's book will create a tide of public opinion about the wonders of water.*"

The Connection Newspaper

"*We have, he says in a new and highly controversial book, Your Body's Many Cries for Water, forgotten how to respond to our numerous thirst signals. But if, instead of taking painkillers and medication, we just drank lots of ordinary tap water, we would probably find that not only the pain, but also the condition would go away for ever.*"

***The Independent*, London, England**

Small Press Selection:

"Your Body's Many Cries for Water, a health book authored by a doctor combining holistic and medical facts about the effects of water and its healing possibilities on many diseases. This book was chosen since water is a topic that has increasing awareness in the marketplace and the author has credentials."

Jan Nathan, Executive Director
Publishers Marketing Association

"Both these books, as well as the publishing firm, bring the sort of news that could change your life. Claims and counter-claims aside, Dr. Batmanghelidj has really got hold of something."

The Book Reader

"Stomach pains, migraines, allergies, asthma, and even arthritis may all be symptoms of dehydration that could easily be cured by a few more glasses of household tap water. But only drinking water when you are feeling thirsty will not provide you with enough, according to F. Batmanghelidj, whose controversial book, Your Body's Many Cries for Water, sold tens of thousands of copies in the United States last year. "

Daily Mail, London, England

Front cover: No pills! No pain! No fooling! ARTHRITIS CURE IN YOUR KITCHEN - Doctor's discovery heals for pennies a day.

National Examiner
December 14, 1993

"Batmanghelidj gives example of patients who have followed his advice using ordinary tap water with positive results in reduction of blood pressure, allergy relief and weight loss. He even goes so far as to link the lack of water with depression."

THE IRISH TIMES

"It does seem sensible to adhere to the logic of the natural and the simple in medicine as fostered in the book, Your Body's Many Cries for Water."

Monsignor Philip A. Gray

"Yours is the most elegant description of arthritic pain I've ever read!"

Perry A. Chapdelaine, Sr., M.A.
Executive Director,
The Arthritis Fund/The Rheumatoid Disease Foundation

Index

Other Health Education Products
by F. Batmanghelidj, M.D
Books

Your Body's Many Cries for Water
The Best-Selling Book
That has Brought Natural Healing to Millions!

This easy-to-read book is your guide to recognizing when your body is calling for water instead of costly prescription drugs (and their dangerous and life-threatening side effects). You'll get a better understanding of how unintentional dehydration is often the root cause of many painful degenerative diseases like asthma, allergies, hypertension, obesity and depression. Among other things, you will learn how to use water to eliminate pain, including heartburn, back pain, arthritis, angina and migraine headaches. Asthma can be cured in a few hours to a few days, naturally and forever. Also, lose weight effortlessly without denying yourself your favorite foods. Learn how to control your blood pressure and cholesterol levels naturally, and prevent sudden heart attacks.

ISBN: 0962994235
Paperback, 200 pages, $14.95
ISBN: 0962994251
Hard cover, 200 pages, $17.00 (retails for $27.00)
Packaging and postage, single book, $5.00

How to Deal with Back Pain and Rheumatoid Joint Pain

This educational, preventive-treatment manual gives you easy-to-use techniques for relieving chronic back pain and rheumatoid joint pain. It's the ideal accompaniment to Dr. Batmanghelidj's video, "How to Deal with Back Pain," since it illustrates and explains the easy-to-do corrective body movements for instant and lasting back pain relief. You will learn the importance of maintaining the proper alkalinity in your body's cells and how water and salt can be used to wash away the acidity that causes pain. You will understand the structure of your body's spinal column, vertebrae and joints – made easy with the book's clearly presented pictures, graphics and model demonstrations. You will also learn simple, everyday techniques for preventing strained muscles, and the important role of the foot and its arches in supporting the body in motion.

ISBN: 09629942-0-0
Paperback, 120 pages, $14.95
Packaging and postage, single book, $5.00

NEW! Water: for Health, for Healing, for Life

Based on more than twenty years of clinical and scientific research into the role of water in the body, Dr. Batmanghelidj shows how water can relieve a stunning range of medical conditions. Simply adjusting your fluid and salt intakes can help you treat and prevent dozens of diseases, avoid costly prescription drugs, and enjoy vibrant new health.

Discover:

- How much water and salt you need each day to stay healthy
- Why other beverages, including tea, coffee, and sodas, cannot be substituted for water
- How to help prevent life-threatening conditions such as heart failure, stroke, Alzheimer's disease, Parkinson's disease, and cancer.
- Why water is the key to losing weight without dieting
- How to hydrate your skin to combat premature aging

ISBN – 9702458-4-X
Hard cover book, 204 pages, $17.00 (retails for $27.00)
Packaging and postage, single book, $5.00

NEW! Water Cures: Drugs Kill

This new book has been compiled to turn conventional medicine on its head. The revelations you'll read here will transform the practice of medicine all over the world. They will change the present cost-intensive, drug peddling, and commerce driven medical system to a physiology-based and disease preventing natural approach to health.

Water Cures: Drugs Kill contains 180 pages of case histories of people for whom the water cure worked. You will read how the conventional drug based medical system failed these people. Dr. B's observations concerning our "sick care" system, as he calls it, are not complementary!

ISBN – 0-9702458-1-5
Paperback, 228 pages, $15.00
Packaging and postage, single book, $5.00

Special Report: Pain: Arthritis Pain & Back Pain

This special report on pain explains the importance of pain as a thirst signal of the body, and why arthritis and back pain are the same dehydration-producing signals that signify a disease-producing level of local drought in different regions of the body.

12 pages, $10.00
Packaging and postage, single report, $5.00

NEW! Los Muchos Clamores de su Cuerpo por Agua

Un preventivo manual autodidáctico para los que prefieren adherirse a la lógica de lo natural y simple. Esta es la primera edición en español del famoso libro del Dr. F.Batmaghalidj. Su mensaje ha sido recibido por millones de personas en todo el mundo, y en muchos idiomas, ahora se ha completado este sueño para él que tiene un escenario de 400 millones de almas. Se recomienda su lectura y además la adopción de sus recomendaciones. No los defraudará. El siempre dice que trabaja para Dios...nuestro creador

ISBN – 0-9702458-3-1
Paperback, 240 pages, $15.00
Packaging and postage, single book, $5.00

Water: Rx for a Healthier, Pain-Free Life

A comprehensive handbook that also serves as a guideline to the information covered in the audio taped presentations itemized below.

For best results, read it before you listen to the tapes. It will prepare your mind so you gain maximum benefit from the information presented in the audiotape seminar. This guide is also an invaluable reference manual to recognizing your body's thirst signals...the common health problems that often result from unintentional dehydration...and how to treat them with the proper timing and correct proportions of water and salt.

50 pages, $7.00
Packaging and postage, single book, $5.00

Videos & DVDs

Cure Pain and Prevent Cancer

Videotaped Presentation at Yoga Research Society 1997 Conference – Thomas Jefferson University Medical School.

Dr. Batmanghelidj explains the link between chronic pain and cancer, and shows you how to use water and salt to relieve pain and prevent disease in this fascinating two-hour videotaped program. In this enlightening presentation, Dr. Batmanghelidj explains how pain is a cry from your body for more water and salt, and is a warning sign that you could be at risk for cancer or other serious illness. New research on how your immune system becomes prone to uncontrolled cell overgrowth, DNA damage and DNA repair dysfunction that leads to cancer shows a vital dependence of your body not just on water, but on salt as well. In fact, a whole host of d3generative diseases are linked not only to dehydration but also to inadequate salt intake.

Dr. Batmanghelidj demonstrates why salt should be taken with water. Learn how to use both water and salt in the proper balance. Learn why pain is a thirst signal you can't afford to ignore! This video helps you recognize your body's emergency calls – and easily missed silent cries – for water. Dr. Batmanghelidj presents his latest research findings and recommendations so you'll know exactly what steps to take to shield yourself and those close to you from pain and disease.

ISBN: 0-9629942-9-4
2 hour, color, VHS, $30.00
DVD, $30.00
Packaging and postage, single item, $5.00

How to Deal with Back Pain

This easy-to-follow program shows you how to promote fluid circulation in your spinal discs to gain instant relief of back pain and sciatic pain. It also exposes the latest scientific breakthroughs on the physiology of chronic back pain. The Video provides step-by-step instructions to help you identify the source and location of your pain. It shows simple body exercises that actually normalize the position of the vertebral discs and draw the pain-causing disc away from the spinal cord to normally relieve sciatic pain within a half hour. The exercises also strengthen the "stays of your spine," back muscles, tendons and ligaments to prevent further suffering.

A safe, doctor-designed approach that has brought soothing, long-lasting comfort to thousands of viewers.

ISBN – 0-9629942-1-9
25 minutes, color, VHS, $29.95
DVD, $29.95
Packaging and postage, single tape, $5.00

Health Miracles in Water & Salt, Choice Medications for Cure of Pain and Disease, Including Cancer

Dr. B's 2-hour plus Medical Yoga 2001 lecture at Thomas Jefferson University Hospital, Department of Integrative Medicine, highlights the important disease-preventing roles of water and salt in the human body. This information represents a medical breakthrough within the science of physiology and openly challenges the sanity and sincerity of the pharmaceutical approach to the treatment of many health problems by the practitioners of conventional medicine.

ISBN 0-9702458-0-7
2 hour, color, VHS, $30.00
Packaging and postage, single tape, $5.00
(Also available as a:
DVD, $30.00, S&H, $5.00
CD set, $20.00, S&H, $5.00
Audio set, $18.00, S&H, $5.00)

NEW! Dehydration and Cancer

This video takes you to Dr. B's 2002-invited lecture at the Cancer Control Society. In the same way the topic of the lecture stunned the audience at the convention, this half-hour video will change how you think about your future health. It will give you the in-depth science behind the benefits of hydration. It will teach you how to protect yourself from asthma, allergies and hypertension; how to gain immediate relief from morning sickness, heartburn, and back pain. It explains how migraine headaches, rheumatoid joint pain of fibromyalgia pain, and indeed, all the major pains of the body denote dehydration where you feel pain. Together, they denote ongoing complications leading to more serious disease. You will understand the roll of pH in wellness, and discover the keys to fighting obesity, Alzheimer's, MS and CANCER, exhaustion, depression and cravings. Learn why, and what you can do to help yourself.

30 minutes, color, VHS or DVD, $20.00
Packaging and postage, single item, $5.00

Audiotapes and CDs

Water: Rx for a Healthier, Pain-Free Life

A comprehensive yet easy-to-understand, 10-hour audio course detailing the role of water and its miraculous healing power.

This comprehensive, 10-hour audiotape seminar gives you a firm foundation for Dr. Batmanghelidj's natural water cure program. You'll get answers to the most frequently asked "whys" and "hows" of the water cure and learn how it can be used to treat a surprisingly broad range of ailments. Dr. Batman explains in detail the body's newly discovered thirst perceptions and crisis signals of dehydration – and why so many "disease conditions" are actually states of dehydration that can be prevented and cured by balancing one's daily water and salt intake. These eight informative audiotapes are ideal for anytime listening – at home, on the road or for group discussions. They are an excellent source of information for the visually impaired.

ISBN: 0-9629942-7-8
8 tape album plus a 50-page guidebook, $67.00
8 CD album plus a 50-page guidebook, $75.00
Packaging and postage, one album, $7.00

Your Body's Many Cries for Water

Lecture at the 39th PA Annual Natural Living Conference at Kutztown University, Kutztown, PA 1993

The lecture got a standing ovation! Learn where and when the water cure was discovered. Learn the way Alexander Fleming discovered penicillin. Learn what he told Dr. Batmanghelidj when he was Sir Alexander's student. Learn why water can permanently erase pain and counteract the effects of stress. Discover the pain-relieving properties of water and why pain is a sign of serious, system-wide dehydration. Learn how you can shut off pain without aspirin, NSAIDS and other side-effect-ridden drugs. You'll be inspired by the real-life examples of people who have used the "watercure" to put an end to their pain and suffering.

90 minutes audio cassette, $10.00,   CD $15.00
Packaging and postage, single item, $5.00

Water: The New Immune Breakthrough & Pain and Cancer "Wonder Drug"

Capital University of Integrative Medicine: Postgraduate Guest Lecture Tape.

In this tape/CD, you will hear what a group of postgraduate health care professionals, including medical doctors and chiropractors, learned about dehydration as the primary cause of the painful degenerative diseases of the human body. This tape/CD contains information on how cancer occurs when there is long-term shortage of water in the body. Two case histories of breast cancer and lymphoma that have gone into remission because of increased water intake are introduced.

95 minutes, $10.00; packaging and postage, single tape, $3.00
Compact Disc, $18.00; packaging and postage, $4.00

Water & Salt: Rx for Total Healing

Tape of Dr. F. Batmanghelidj's opening address at 1999 Pennsylvania Annual Natural Living Conference, Cedar Crest College Allentown, PA

90 minutes, audio cassette $10.00, CD $15.00
Packaging and postage, single item, $5.00

Multiple Sclerosis: Is "Water" Its Cure?

Real-life Evidence of the Link between Dehydration and MS.

In this lively audiotape of the "Just Common Sense" radio program hosted by Bob Butts, you will hear from a young male MS sufferer who used Dr. Batman's water and salt program to put an end to his symptoms. This revealing interview with Dr. Batman explains how you can use the same water and salt cure to bring relief to the incapacitating fatigue, swelling and vision and cognitive problems that plague MS sufferers. He also discusses the destructive effects of caffeine on memory and energy.

69 minutes, audio cassette $10.00, CD $15.00
Packaging and postage, single item, $5.00

New: December 2004

Obesity Cancer Depression:
Their Common Cause & Natural Cure

The Wisdom of Water
Preventing Dehydration Prevents Serious Diseases

·   Learn why—to avoid getting fat, becoming depressed and
    developing cancer—water should be your #1 dietary supplement.

·   Discover how water stimulates the enzymes that burn fat and
    permanently reduce weight—30-50 pounds without any effort.

·   Discover how water manufactures hydroelectric energy in ever
    cell of your body, reducing your need to constantly eat food.

·   Discover why your brain prefers the "clean energy from water"
    than the "dirty energy from food."

·   Discover how most people get fat because they confuse thirst
    with hunger.

·   Discover how water makes your brain work like an atomic clock,
    restores your enthusiasm, and fills you with the joys of life—the
    sunny side of you.

·   Discover how water is your natural anticancer medication.

·   Discover how dehydration suppresses the immune system in the
    bone marrow, whereas proper hydration maximizes the immune
    system activity.

·   Discover how water and salt can actually send killer cancers into
    remission, for years—the medical norm for a cure.

Paperback; 240 pages
ISBN 0-9702458-2-3;
$15.00
Packaging and postage, single book, $5.00

To order the above items, send check or money order to:

Global Health Solutions
P.O. Box 3189
Falls Church, Va. 22043
Tel. 703-848-2333, Fax: 703-848-0028

Discount given for orders of five or more books
VISA, MasterCard and Discover orders only:
1-800-759-3999

VA State tax should be added to orders by Virginia residents

Or order on our website:
Website address: www.watercure.com

Personal Notes